The Benzo Devil

The Benzo Devil

How I Recovered From Prescription Drugs

R.W. PHARAZYN

IMPORTANT NOTICE:

Any information given in this book should not be substituted for the advice of a physician who is well informed about benzodiazepine addiction and withdrawal. All information given here is opinion only and therefore is to be followed at your own risk. Abrupt cessation of benzodiazepines may be very dangerous. Always consult your prescriber if you are considering making any changes.

Please read the complete disclaimer at the end of this book relating to all the content and advice within.

*This book is dedicated to
first and foremost
Emeritus Professor Heather Ashton.
Also, a tilt to Peter Edge, Leisurely
Richard, Ray King, Margie, Captain
Mkrl (for his constant encouragement),
Gabe and Deke plus all the divinely
damaged of this world.*

Contents

Introduction   1

Part I. My Personal Story

1. Childhood and education   9

2. My benzo background   16

3. Radio days and panic attacks   20

4. My introduction to Ativan   24

5. Talkback radio king   29

6. Doctors and bad choices   35

7. All hell broke loose   41

8. Upon reflection   46

9. The 'shrink'   50

10. London calling   57

11. Prescription reality check in Clapham   61

12. Fleeing back to Australia   68

Part II. Waltzing with the Devil, Narcotics
Anonymous and Withdrawal

13.   In off the deep end   79

14.   The self-detox fallout   84

15.   Now for the crazy stuff   89

16.   My 'shrink' betrays me   94

17.   Cuckoo's nest and golden beaches   100

18.   Hallucinations, poodles and dolphins   107

19.   Madness, counsellors and suicide   113

20.   Narcotics Anonymous to the rescue   121

21.   Brother Red and the Na-Na meetings   128

22.   Was my life ruined by benzos?   132

23.   Nimbin, pythons and synchronicity   137

24.   Time to move forward on the quest   145

25.   Giving something back   149

26.   Taking that next big step   156

27.   Family ... what family?   162

28.   Baby steps to recovery   166

29.   Transcendental meditation   173

Part III. Into the Light

30.   Case studies of benzo sadness   183

31. The arrival of the cavalry   187

32. Tangling with bureaucracy   193

33. Medical misadventure?   199

34. Back to work   206

35. Becoming Rupert Murdoch?   212

36. Romance and little critters   216

37. Fortune, fame and The Golden Dawn   219

38. The big payoff   225

39. Roaming the world after recovery   231

40. Was it all worth it?   234

41. The last hurrah   239

Part IV. The Facts

42. Background information   245

43. Emeritus Professor Heather Ashton   248

44. Why should you come off   252
     benzodiazepines?

45. Before starting benzo withdrawal   255

46. The withdrawal   261

47. Stepping into freedom   274

48. Long-term effects of benzodiazepines   276

49. Recurrence of symptoms after successful   278
     withdrawal

50. The end, the last tango   *283*

References and links   *285*
Disclaimer   *288*
About the Author   *290*

Introduction

Bernard also laughed; after two grams of soma the joke seemed, for some reason, good. Laughed and then, almost immediately, dropped off to sleep.
— Aldous Huxley, *Brave New World*

Seventies-era rock star Stevie Nicks of superstar band Fleetwood Mac is the poster girl for the perils of benzodiazepine addiction. In almost every interview, the former lead singer of Fleetwood Mac makes a point of mentioning the toll her abuse of the prescription drug has taken on her life.

While promoting her solo album *In Your Dreams*, she told Fox News that she blamed benzodiazepines for the fact that she never had children.

'The only thing I'd change [in my life] is walking into the office of that psychiatrist who prescribed me Klonopin. That ruined my life for eight years,' she said. 'God knows, maybe I would have met someone, maybe I would have had a baby.'

Nicks has described the benzo drugs as a 'horrible, dangerous drug', and said that her eventual 45-day hospital detox and rehab from the drug felt like 'somebody opened up a door and pushed me into hell'.

Professor Malcolm H Lader, Royal Maudsley Hospital, BBC Radio 4, 'Face the Facts':

'It is more difficult to withdraw people from benzodiazepines than it is from heroin. It just seems that the dependency is so ingrained and the withdrawal symptoms you get are so intolerable, that people have a great deal of problems coming off. The other aspect is that with heroin, usually the withdrawal is over within a week or so. With benzodiazepines, a proportion of patients go on to long–term withdrawal and they have very unpleasant symptoms for month after month, and I get letters from people saying you can go on for two years or more. Some of the tranquilliser groups can document people who still have symptoms ten years after stopping.'

The former UK Prime Minister David Cameron on benzodiazepine addiction, 2013:

'Firstly, I pay tribute to the Honourable Gentleman [Jim Dobbin, MP], who has campaigned strongly on this issue over many years. He is right to say that this is a terrible affliction; these people are not drug addicts but they have become hooked on repeat prescriptions of tranquillisers. The Minister for Public Health is very happy to discuss this issue with him and, as he says, make sure that the relevant guidance can be issued.'

Benzodiazepines were discovered, more or less by chance, by a Dr Sternbach, working for Hoffman-La Roche pharmaceutical company in New Jersey, USA. In 1957, the original compound was found to have hypnotic, anxiolytic (anxiety-reducing) and muscle relaxant effects, and the first benzodiazepine, chlordiazepoxide (Librium), was launched in the UK in 1960, followed by diazepam (Valium) in 1963.

Valium became the first 'blockbuster' drug. During its peak year of sales, 1978, Americans consumed 2.3 billion Valium tablets. It was the single most prescribed drug in the USA from 1969 until 1982, and was, according to a press release from Roche, 'the largest-selling, pharmaceutical in the world'. Its sales helped make Roche a giant in the pharmaceutical industry.

Having relinquished his rights to his employer, Dr Leo Sternbach was paid a royalty of US$1.00 on the patent for the drug in his name. He didn't like taking Valium himself, claiming it made him feel 'depressed', which is somewhat ironic.

By 1983, there were 17 benzodiazepines on the market, earning the drug companies nearly US$3 billion worldwide, annually. There are now 29 benzodiazepines available in Europe, the USA, UK, Australasia and most of the developed countries.

Riding high on such a global money-spinner came the introduction of the new Z-drugs. Zopiclone (introduced in 1998), Zolpidem and Zaleplon (in 2000), and now Eszopiclone (in 2005) were the main ones prescribed by doctors around the world. They act like benzodiazepines and are generally prescribed for sleep problems. Then, of course, there are the highly addictive prescription opioids, like methadone and oxycodone, which are two of the most overdosed drugs out there, killing 14,000 Americans in 2014 alone, including sending a fair swathe of celebrities, such as Heath Ledger, to the Pearly Gates.

Between 1999 and 2014, sales of prescription opioid

drugs almost quadrupled in the US, an increase that came not simply in response to patient suffering but because more of the population are addicted to these powerful drugs. Such is the demand for them, Americans now consume four-fifths of the global supply (*The Economist*, 6 April 2017).

There is no perfect time to give up an addiction

It's taken me a long time to get down and write this book, as it brings up so many dark memories that I've found it easier to simply let sleeping dogs lie and file my incredible journey as something best forgotten. But here it is, the second decade of the 21st century, so I have decided, in the interests of millions of people around the world who are still addicted to prescription drugs, to go back to the nineties where the path to a drug-free recovery began for me. I hope that my experiences might give those of you addicted to benzodiazepines some solace and courage to break free from this chemical curse.

Writing a book advocating that those people trapped in an addiction to prescription drugs should follow my path into detoxification, withdrawal and eventual recovery didn't seem to me to be something that was worth doing, unless I could actually show that the whole process was positively life-changing and that I had personally achieved a happy ending, proving that there was, indeed, life after addiction. But, yes, I got my happy ending and it was well worth the journey, so here I am writing the book and, no, it's not a 'misery memoir'.

My story is divided into four parts. The first part up to chapter 12 is my personal back story and the path my earlier life took which would eventually lead me into a dependency/addiction to benzodiazepine tranquillisers. In the second and most gruelling part up to chapter 29, I recount for you in stark and vivid detail my experience of all the hellish days of self-detox, withdrawal and borderline madness, and then in the third part up to chapter 41, eventual salvation and clarity in my new drug-free world. Finally, in Part Four, following the end of my personal story, I go into comprehensive detail, mainly based on protocols outlined in recognised research, about withdrawal methods, help agencies and website links, etc. so if you want to get clean from prescription drugs of any kind, you will have plenty of information and support mechanisms and you won't be alone, as I was.

When I started into self-detox and withdrawal in the nineties, there was virtually nothing available to assist and guide me through that dreadful process. The medical profession was only into prescribing benzos and very few mainstream doctors had much, if any, knowledge on how to go about entering the process of withdrawal from tranquillisers. Hopefully, my book will help to give you the inspiration and knowledge that a better, brighter life awaits you and will provide you with a clear map for you to follow on the rocky path to freedom.

Good luck! It will be worth it.

PART I

My Personal Story

1

Childhood and education

He who rides the tiger, finds it difficult to dismount.
— Rudyard Kipling

My name is Rob Pharazyn and this is my story.

In the early nineties, I limped back from Australia to my home country of New Zealand, emotionally and physically shattered.

All I wanted to do was to put back together the broken pieces of my life and try to forget what I had been through in my quest for freedom from my 13-year dependency on benzodiazepine prescription tranquillisers.

I had very little money left, was unemployed, on a sickness benefit and living in a rented bedsitter at a downmarket boarding house, which was certainly a long way from the lifestyle to which I had previously been accustomed.

After struggling to get occasional work and coming to terms with the fact that my life was probably over in any measurable sense and existing in quiet despair, a strange turn of events occurred which changed my future.

It was as if the gods had looked down and decided, 'We can't break him so stamp his hand and let him through!'

The metaphoric cavalry had arrived for me and from that point onwards, I never looked back. I'll tell you all about it as we navigate our way through this book with despair and sometimes amusement, but we now need to start at the beginning of my life for reasons that will become obvious.

I think there was always a certain, but not unusual, synchronistic destiny attached to the path that would lead me to take my very first round of prescription 'benzos'.

I was brought up by middle- to upper-class parents in Nelson, New Zealand. Parents who really had no clear knowledge of giving love to a child and who also had their own fair share of dysfunctionality in their preceding family tree. In hindsight, I can see genetic dispositions towards anxiety, whether hereditary or induced, amongst my various family members.

I say this because modern genetics and neuroscience point towards a potential anxiety gene running through some families as a hereditary factor and to the likelihood within such families of some members ending up using a crutch for anxiety relief, be it drugs or alcohol.

In my case, emotional deprivation as a child and the words 'happy, healthy bonding' weren't part of my personal lexicon and the results of this emotional starvation were to become apparent as I grew into adulthood.

We don't choose our family, so when talking about my childhood, I do agree with Johann Hari, author of the 2016 *New York Times* bestselling book *Chasing the Scream: The First* and *Last Days of the War on Drugs*, that if we don't get early childhood love, then we are on a likely collision course for an addiction to something, somewhere down the track.

'Human beings have a natural and innate need to bond. And when we're happy and healthy, we'll bond and connect with each other,' Hari explains. *'But if you can't do that because you're traumatised or isolated or beaten down by life you will bond with something that will give you some sense of relief, be it drugs, alcohol, porn or gambling.'*

In my upbringing, a gentleman alcoholic father and a neurotic mother were my parental role models. I don't recall any demonstrations of physical or emotional affection towards me by either of them and really can't remember ever having any guidance or meaningful conversations with my father or mother. She was a highly creative but equally highly-strung woman who was either fun or foe, depending on the day, and my father was simply too weak emotionally to shoulder any responsibility for my upbringing.

In fairness to him, he'd never known parental love, having been brought up by nannies (governess), as my grandparents were very wealthy dissolutes who had no idea about children and had raised him along the English, upper-class model. Poor bastard didn't stand a chance really!

To grow up with no template of what love from a parent feels like is not a good thing for any child. I can only now, as an adult, imagine how different things may have turned out for me under a more loving and capable set of parental circumstances.

But whether it was a genetic or deficient upbringing by my parents, or just that I was a rebel without a cause as I approached my teens, the end result was that my default setting was to be continually kicking against the system.

I was always railing against the facile 'one size fits all' disciplines and impositions made upon me at my upmarket boarding school and by society in general.

Boarding schools were often where parents sent their children when they couldn't figure out how to handle their child's upbringing. In my instance, Nelson College (which was where I was sent) was founded in 1857 and modelled along the same lines as the old English schools, such as Rugby and Eton. I was just over 10 years old when I was thrown in as a preparatory pupil amongst bullies, prefects, perverts and sadistic masters, where constant caning and punishment were the order of the day. I wept daily, riddled with homesickness, for the first two weeks after my arrival so they moved me to a different inter-collegiate 'house' where my older brother was, with the supposed benefit being that his proximity would calm me down and make me feel happier. He never spoke to me because he was three years senior to me and I was also promptly molested at night, after lights out, by an older boy in the dormitory bed next to me. At that age, I didn't even know what masturbation was. Welcome to the jungle, Rob!

It's not hard to see how much that would affect a young boy's formative years and although I was by no means alone or even singled out, I know it damaged me. If ever a tendency towards anxiety was going to be formed, it was there.

My early 'fight or flight' switch was set on 'high' far too early in my childhood, so my cortisol levels were probably constantly marinating on red alert. All my days as a junior boy at college were spent in apprehension that some senior boy or prefect was going to pull me aside and make me recite the college song, the rugby chant, what was written under the sundial or any number of litanies that you'd been forced to learn by rote from day one of arriving at the school. Failure to be word perfect would result in a beating with a cane, or worse.

They had a system which gave prefects or masters the right to give you a 'fatigue', which was rather like an on-the-spot fine. Every Saturday morning, the fatigue list would be posted with the jobs you had to do as punishment. If you accrued three or more fatigues in a week, you not only had to do the jobs on the list, but also got a caning from a master, so you had the whole week to build up your anxiety levels till the list was posted and your beating arrived.

It was not uncommon to be sound asleep after dormitory lights went out, to suddenly be hauled out of bed for a mass caning in your pyjamas because someone amongst the boys in the dormitory had been committing the cardinal sin of talking after lights out!

At 13 years of age, I ran away, absconded, went over the wall, fled.

Call it what you like, I just wanted to not be there. Two other boarders had done the same thing, but had glamorised their escape by stealing a car only to be caught, expelled and criminally convicted. I raised the bar in the glamour stakes by catching a bus, and after a few days 'on the run', I was picked up by the cops whilst hitchhiking along a main highway, shivering my butt off, as it was the middle of the New Zealand winter. For my crime, I was given six whippings on my backside with the cane and put into what was known as 'Coventry', which is a quaint old boarding school custom whereby for the next two weeks, for the sin of bringing the college into disrepute, absolutely no one was permitted to speak to me under any circumstances.

This suited me just fine and I enjoyed the peace and the disdain. We can all be heroes, if just for one day!

I've tried to go back and cognitively re-label some of the things that happened at boarding school but it's just too far back and too deep in my psyche to reach and label it for what it really was. Cruelty! Dysfunctional parents and being thrown into an institution for six years where pain and punishment lurked everywhere from the moment you opened your eyes at 6am on a frosty morning till when you went to bed and the lights went out, pretty much set me up to always be on constant guard and, I guess, become future anxiety-damaged goods. Maybe, maybe not?

At 17, I left college with good academic qualifications allowing me into university, but after being incarcerated at my alma mater since I was just a child, the last thing I wanted was more study and dull living. My parents had finally given up on each other and were now going through a divorce at the same time as my leaving college, so they were preoccupied with their own misery. I sprang up like an uncaged animal and seized life by the throat, literally going for it, free of all restrictions and following the fun trail with my main drug of choice up until my early twenties being alcohol, party, girls, party.

It's interesting looking back on my youth with the benefit of adult experience and hindsight. At the time, you're just hanging on to the end of the racing car known as your life, not thinking too much about the indicators in your behaviour. Now, as an older man, I can see that I was probably a bit of a troubled soul, masking certain anxieties with alcohol as many others in my cohort were doing at that age.

2

My benzo background

The era was the late sixties, early seventies and, as is the wont of the young, no one thought much about underlying causes for our actions, just perpetual fun.

We had all laughed along with The Rolling Stones when they had hit songs on the radio about 'Mother's little helper' and the '19th nervous breakdown' which were, of course, about suburban neurosis and the stay-at-home housewives swallowing tranquillisers to dampen down the nibbling anxiety and Lucy Jordanesque madness that threatened to come in from the boundaries of their minds to swamp them as they led their quietly desperate lives in the suburbs, washing babies' nappies and waiting for their husbands to return from work.

Simultaneously, in those swinging sixties, the prescription benzos, like Librium and Valium, had appeared as if by magic around the world, courtesy of the drug companies, and were being handed out like lollies by well-meaning GPs.

'Sorry, Mrs Jones, I can only spare ten minutes so take some of these, come back next month and we'll see how you're settling into the cooking and washing those nappies. Oh, and say hi to Mr Jones from me, won't you?'

The first wave of what was eventually to turn into a drug tsunami and create hundreds of millions of drug dependants was being hatched globally. In fairness to the doctors of that era, I suspect that back then the dispensing of the benzodiazepine family of drugs was originally done with the best of intentions by naïve doctors and pharmacists. The world was a different place and possibly more well meaning than it is today, so a lot of doctors probably thought they were helping, rather than creating addicted suburban zombies amongst their patients, by dishing out without question this 'shiny, new wonder drug' called Valium.

Coming on the back of the advent of the contraceptive pill and drugs such as LSD and the whole hippie/free love explosion, the prescribing of a chill pill that appeared to work probably didn't seem like such a bad thing at the time.

But the evil genie was now out of the bottle and it never stopped morphing into the monster it eventually became. Like a runaway train, it grew and grew until now, here in the South Pacific where I reside, huge numbers of Australians and New Zealanders swallow a wide range of available benzodiazepines.

According to prescription statistics, nearly two million people just in Australasia have taken benzodiazepines every day for months, years, sometimes a lifetime. In the United States of America, over 100 million prescriptions are written each year for any one of the benzodiazepines such as Ativan, Valium and Xanax, with Xanax being the most popular drug of all time.

There's no doubt that when first taken, benzos do a fine job of calming the nervous system and cutting back anxiety, but any longer than two to four weeks and you're potentially addicted to their actions. It's that simple.

It seems that they work by enhancing the transmission of a naturally occurring chemical in the brain called GABA (gamma-aminobutyric acid), which depresses activity in the part of the brain that controls emotions. More GABA equals less stress until your brain stops producing the natural GABA and the substitute chemical benzo version kicks in. Voila! Another addict is born.

Coincidentally, benzos are also prescribed to relax damaged muscles after sporting injuries, car accident fallout or back pain, which is proof that you don't have to be crazy to take them. However, a lot of sporting people without any anxiety issues have also struggled with chronic detox and equally horrific withdrawal symptoms when trying to stop taking the dreaded benzos.

It seems hard to believe that, despite suspicions about the long-term risks being raised only a couple of years after the first benzos came on the market in the sixties, no notice of these warnings was taken by the medical profession. Throughout the seventies when tranquilliser use was really starting to take off, clinical papers about addiction and withdrawal appeared in medical journals and by 1980 there was clear evidence emerging that on normal, prescribed doses of a benzodiazepine, no matter the brand name, one in three patients who took the drug for more than a few weeks or months at the most, suffered acute withdrawal when they tried to cease taking the drug.

But still doctors kept handing them out like there was no tomorrow, creating an army of unwitting addicts, as is still the case to this very day.

3

Radio days and panic attacks

Back now to my own personal glide path to a pilled-out Armageddon.

In my early twenties, I found myself in Brisbane, Australia, living the high life and eventually marrying a woman who, at the time, I thought I loved. My wife was beautiful, my friends were everywhere and I was on top of my game. Then the Fates stepped in and my world slowly but surely started to spin off its axis. The karmic wheel was now preparing me for future circumstances that were to suck me down into the eventual darkness of the abyss of prescription drug withdrawal.

After a relatively short duration, my marriage flew to pieces and I experienced for the first time in my life, real crushing sadness, anxiety and probably reactive depression. Many of you reading this book will be able to relate to just how hard it is to contend with the sense of failure of a marital break-up, and although my ex-wife and I had a couple of shots at reconciliation, we eventually called it a day and went our separate ways.

Up until this period of my life, most of my employment had revolved around the arena of sales and marketing and I had built up a good CV working for large, multinational companies ranging from EMI Recording to Gillette, etc. but in the wreckage of my marriage, the antidote to the pain became clear to me.

I turned my back on all that I'd known in the executive work scene.

I ran away and became a radio disc jockey!

It seemed like the perfect place to 'hide' and, at the time, I was good friends with two of New Zealand's top radio jocks, so with a little help from my friends, I was skilled up and by surreptitious means I found myself behind the microphone doing my first on-air gig at a station called Radio Windy in Wellington, New Zealand.

Like millions around the globe, I was a big fan of the now deceased David Bowie. He was successfully playing with his persona, turning up in different guises from his first incarnation of Ziggy Stardust to The Thin White Duke, so I figured that I would do the same with Rob Pharazyn on the radio and it worked like a charm. Goodbye, unhappy marriage and failure; hello, Mr DJ.

I springboarded in a very short time from late nights on Radio Windy, New Zealand, to the high-powered world of Australian radio, criss-crossing over a couple of smaller radio stations until I beat the odds by ending up on top Sydney station, 2UW. Sydney is Australia's biggest and most glittering city. Rob Pharazyn the radio man was really pumping now with lots of record company promo parties, free weed, Veuve champagne, etc. along with accommodating young women, which all went towards cementing the ego and self-image nicely in place.

After my time in Australia, I returned to New Zealand, a fully–fledged, competent and skilled radio jock, and soon found myself doing a prime-time morning shift on a southern city rock station: 3ZM in Christchurch. At that time, we were one of the first stations to use computers to programme the music as announce-assist and the pressure was on. I was pumping the music, the fan mail was coming in and my nights were taken up with smoking dope, listening to bands at local clubs and being the man about town. But, like a distant drum and not so deep down, the ghosts in that nagging old subconscious were rising up ever more frequently, commandeered by the 'bitch with the whip', to persecute and frighten me as they demanded attention to their negative whisperings of failed marriage, low self-esteem and all the other usual suspects. "That persona thing might've worked for David Bowie, but it ain't gonna work for you, sonny boy."

One morning, after a particularly hard night and severely hungover, I was on-air talking live to the city whilst at the same time, during the music sweeps, recording an off-air interview on another channel with the members of the band Talking Heads, coming to me from a loft somewhere in New York City. They also had Brian Eno and Jonathan Richman from the Modern Lovers with them, so it was a very frisky interview. They were promoting their forthcoming New Zealand tour but in between my questions, I was busily throwing up in the studio rubbish tin, due to the combo of a raspberry milkshake and too much of everything the night before. When it was all recorded and 'in the can', I rang the station content director upstairs and told him I was ill and had to go home. As I walked to my car, a terrible feeling of fear swept over me and the whole world seem to buckle. For seconds, I had no idea where I was, as everything seemed to distort around me, but I simply put it down to the hangover and got myself together.

The next morning, just before going on-air, I had gone to a cafe near the radio station to get a takeout coffee and was waiting to cross at the traffic lights, when it happened again. Suddenly, and from nowhere, the same feeling of absolute dread and fear consumed me and my brain seemed to seize up completely. My heart felt like it was leaping out of my chest, my head seemed as if it was on fire and I literally couldn't breathe.

I thought I must have been having a heart attack as I stood at the traffic lights hanging on to the pole and probably looking very strange to the surge of people crossing the street, but in reality, this was my first panic attack.

After a few minutes of mental chaos, I settled back down and went on and did my air shift and then made an appointment with a random doctor at some medical clinic that I found in the phone book.

Big, big mistake, and the beginning of my life-changing experience.

4

My introduction to Ativan

I often wonder how things would've panned out if I hadn't made that appointment with an unknown doctor at a clinic that was basically like a drive-through Kentucky Fried Chicken version of medical advice.

It was one of those fast-turnaround prescription type places with no apparent interest in anything more than giving you the basic 10 minutes to find out what your problem was before sending you on your way with a script for some drug in your hot little hand.

The doctor I was allocated to briefly listened to my tale of a rock'n'roll lifestyle and my trouble with what I called 'the speeding brain' syndrome, which meant I spent most nights wide awake trying to shut down my thoughts when endeavouring to get to sleep. When I told him about the panic experiences of the previous days, he casually informed me that I was probably suffering from anxiety-related stress, so the choices I had were to either give up my job or take some pills that he'd prescribe for me. Giving up my job was not on the cards, as the alternative to that was going back to nothing in my mind, and anyway, 'what the hell, everyone's popping some type of pill these days', be they contraceptives or aspirin.

So, I wandered off to a nearby pharmacy and got my prescription filled. On that day in the history of my life, I started the rapid process towards becoming an accidental addict to pills prescribed to me by a medical doctor. Talk about a chemical marriage. Unfortunately, this was to turn out not to be one of those that are blessed in heaven.

The label on the packet told me that my new-found friend was a drug called Ativan (or lorazepam, its generic pharmaceutical name) and I was to take a one milligram tab, three times a day. To my innocent brain, 1mg didn't seem much, and it was only quite a few years later that I found out that part of the shell game the drug companies play is that 1mg of Ativan is equivalent to 10mg of Valium and so the variable goes around, disguised in the different types of benzo brands being dispensed. Some brands were 5mg but really 20mg comparable to similar other types of tranquillisers, etc.

Back then, neither the doctor I saw nor the pharmacist thought it necessary to warn me that this class of drugs potentially had savagely addictive properties and should only be used for a maximum of six weeks to avoid getting hooked.

Would I have still taken them if I had been warned of their addictive properties? Definitely not! No way, Jose! I would've searched for other alternatives.

We've all been brought up from childhood to trust doctors. We have been taught that physicians all swear to the Hippocratic Oath, the most important tenet being *Primum nihil nocere*, which is Latin for 'Above all, do no harm'. Every night on TV, we see advertisements for medicines with the tag phrase 'ask your doctor if this medication is right for you'.

We hear this phrase so often that 'ask your doctor' has the brainwashing effect of instilling complete faith in whatever the doctor tells you is best for you. However, a basic premise of ethical medical practice is what is known as 'informed consent'. Ethically, a doctor should present a patient with the facts concerning an offered treatment or procedure, spelling out the various dangers as well as the possible benefits, and the patient then makes, hopefully, reasoned personal and medical decisions based upon that information. Not to disclose the full risks of substances such as benzodiazepine drugs is not merely uninformed consent but is actually misinformed consent for patients and borders on malpractice, in my opinion. If I had been told that what I was being prescribed would create a potential chemical addiction within as short a space of time as three weeks, I would never have taken them.

To give you an idea of what I was prescribed on that day without any medical advice, here's an official medical breakdown of side effects that are possible from taking the benzo drug Ativan.

Most adverse reactions to benzodiazepines, including CNS effects and respiratory depression, are dose dependent, with more severe effects occurring with high doses.

In a sample of about 3500 patients treated for anxiety, the most frequent adverse reaction to Ativan (lorazepam) was sedation (15.9%), followed by dizziness (6.9%), weakness (4.2%), and unsteadiness (3.4%). The incidence of sedation and unsteadiness increased with age.

Other adverse reactions to benzodiazepines, including lorazepam (Ativan) are fatigue, drowsiness, amnesia, memory impairment, confusion, disorientation, depression, unmasking of depression, disinhibition, euphoria, suicidal ideation/ attempt, ataxia, asthenia, extrapyramidal symptoms, convulsions/seizures tremor, vertigo, eye-function/visual disturbance (including diplopia and blurred vision), dysarthria/ slurred speech, change in libido, impotence, decreased orgasm, headache, coma, respiratory depression, apnoea, worsening of sleep apnoea, worsening of obstructive pulmonary disease, gastrointestinal symptoms including nausea, change in appetite, constipation.

Paradoxical reactions, including anxiety, excitation, agitation, hostility, aggression, rage, sleep disturbances/insomnia, sexual arousal, and hallucinations may occur. Small decreases in blood pressure and hypotension may occur but are usually not clinically significant, probably being related to the relief of anxiety produced by Ativan (lorazepam).

This is obviously a worst-case scenario and I didn't experience all of those outlined symptoms, but I can recognise about 75% on the list, which I experienced in varying degrees over the 13 years of addiction to Ativan.

The major drug companies that manufacture the benzodiazepine group of drugs have a lot to answer for but, in my opinion, the fault can be laid more squarely at the doorstep of the medical profession. Those doctors who prescribe these pills without giving patient advice and then go on prescribing them to the same patient, month after month, year after year are the most culpable and have the most to answer for. In all my time over the 13 years of being hooked on Ativan, I had only one doctor question my usage but none ever refused to give me repeat prescriptions and being in radio, I moved around quite a bit so there were many, different doctors that I visited to get my little white pills.

5

Talkback radio king

So, there we have it. The beginning of the end that would take me through the door into the 'valley of the dolls' of addiction and drug dependency.

I started on the pills as prescribed, taking one in the morning around breakfast, one in the mid-afternoon and one before going to bed at night and, at first, they worked, but within a month, I noticed a lessening effect, which seemed to be replaced by a slight but constant irritability. I followed this daily 3mg regime for the whole 13 years that I was using Ativan, convinced that I wasn't an addict because I wasn't taking any more than the daily recommended dose. But as I pointed out before, unbeknownst to me, I was taking the equivalent of 30 milligrams of Valium a day, which would be considered quite a solid dose.

I'm sorry if I'm already tangling your head up with details, but I know that as well as the many people who wish to know about these drugs, there are a lot of you out there who are reading this who will still be addicted to any one of the multitude of benzo tranquillisers, so it is important you get that dose thing sorted in your head before you even entertain going into a withdrawal or detox regime.

To try giving up without understanding all the facts is a very dangerous move. I'll point you later in part four of this book, to a variety of sources online that can easily clarify the facts behind whatever rubbish drug they've got you on so you can follow a safe withdrawal protocol.

Anyway, there I was rocking along on the radio at 3ZM in Christchurch, New Zealand, taking my pills, and for a while things seemed to settle down and I pretty much forgot about them, other than to take them every day, and they soon became just another background part of my daily carousel of life. A few months later, I moved north to spend nearly three years in paradise living by the seaside in the sunny Bay of Plenty, New Zealand, and successfully programming the music on the local radio station whilst managing a team of happy, young radio jocks. The radio lifestyle naturally involved smoking the local ganja, drinking lots of cold beers and having as much fun as possible. Living *la vida loca* was what it was all about.

In 1982, I and the then love of my life, who also worked with me, decided it was time to give up the good times of sun, sea and rock music at the radio station and move north to Auckland, which is New Zealand's biggest city. For the previous seven years, I'd been involved in music radio as a radio jock and content director, but now my arrival in Auckland saw me take a complete change of direction and I became the evening talkback host on the Radio Pacific network. This was a remarkable experience and in a short space of time I'd built up a strong following throughout the city and around New Zealand. As you can imagine, talking non-stop for four hours to a barrage of callers wanting to rant about everything from incest to life in prison was a very tough challenge to my soul and psyche, and after nearly 12 months of a nightly, relentless ear-bashing, I started getting a return of the mini anxiety attacks while on-air. Not regularly, but suddenly out of the blue on certain nights during an incoming call I'd experience that old, familiar feeling of dread creeping over me for no apparent reason other than the occasional bomb threat or abuse that came with the job.

I'm sure my panel operator never quite knew why I'd sometimes cut short a call and tell him to play some music whilst I threw off my headphones and went for a quick walk around the corridors until I got my head back together. If you can picture having headphones clasped to your skull for four hours as a blitzkrieg of callers washed across your mind, you may be able to understand the intensity of what it was like being in such a situation when the sweat breaks out on your brow and the incoming caller literally stops making sense. On full-moon nights, the calls would become crazier than usual and, as an example, I had one regular caller who would call me up on such a night from his bolt hole somewhere in the city to describe to me and my silent listeners the curious process of shedding his skin and turning into a snake!

'Give me your tired, your poor, your huddled masses yearning to breathe free' and chances are they'll also turn out to be talkback followers (apologies to the Statue of Liberty poem).

However, that was just part of the usual nightly circus and I'd become used to it, but this growing anxiety manifestation puzzled me because, as far as I was concerned, I was taking a daily drug which was meant to prevent this from happening. But as I was to find out some years later, it was the drug that I was taking which was causing the anxious feelings and had long since lost its original purpose, which was to control any anxiety! I can't emphasise this paradoxical fact enough.

The discovery that benzos in a short time of usage potentially start to mirror the original anxiety symptoms that they were prescribed to prevent, was the absolute pivotal, major breakthrough that eventually precipitated my finally taking the plunge and starting the long journey into hell and back to successfully give up taking Ativan. But I'll get to that later.

I should've been on top of the world. By now, I was on the front cover of *Metro*, the number one magazine in the city, yet inside I was starting to very slowly disassemble as the public persona of talkback king and the real Rob Pharazyn battled it out for control, ably abetted by my daily dose of Ativan, acting as destroyer and referee. And, of course, on top of that there was always too much good living of wine, weed and crayfish in the mix as well. (crayfish? what are they doing in this tale? Never mind.)

Most nights, over four hours, I could take around 40 incoming calls whilst out there in the velvet silence of the night, up to 100,000 people (according to ratings surveys) would tune in to sample various parts of my show, so I knew it was more than just the 'orchestra' of the callers that I was conducting my nightly 'symphony' for. Pressure, under pressure!

With surveys showing my popularity still growing, I was

sitting in the studio one night with the calls pouring in. The on-air red light was glowing away as I listened to a caller trying to justify having sex with his daughter. I looked across through the tinted, studio glass window at my young panel operator smiling away at me from the control room. A full rack of call-waiting lights was blinking at me like sinners in a confessional box queuing up to talk to the priest (and I'm not even a Catholic) and at that crucial moment, I thought to myself, 'I just can't do this any more. I can't listen to this rabble of well-intentioned or deluded mish-mash of human beings any longer. I don't care what the cost is … I've got to stop this!'

I've often wondered how it would've all worked out if I'd been in the identical scenario as the successful talkback 'king', but hadn't been taking the benzos, given my later discovery that they were the problem, keeping the anxiety percolating by mirroring my original symptoms. Would the 'Princess' (my lovely girlfriend who worked with me as a newsreader) and I gone on to be the toast of the city and enjoy all the fruits of success that a top-rating radio host would enjoy? Would I have got married and had 2.5 cleanly scrubbed children whilst the Princess and I basked in the sun, sipping Mojitos by our celebrity-sized swimming pool and travelling the world? Probably, but I'll never know because when I finished my shift that night I put together a handwritten resignation and slipped it under the door of the manager of the radio station and went home with my lady, feeling as if a great weight had been lifted off my shoulders.

All hell broke loose the next day with the station management calling me in and reporters pestering me for the reasons as to why I'd chosen to do what no one ever does in the entertainment game, which was to resign when your ratings are going *up*! That's right! The bi-annual survey of all stations had just come out and I had increased my existing personal number one market share by a further 5%, which was an excellent result, but to me it signified that the barbarians at the gate were getting stronger and the nightly madness would only get more suffocating.

Management asked me what they had to do to get me to stay so I gave them a list of outrageous requirements, most of which I knew and hoped they'd never meet. One that I was serious about was that I wanted them to install softly lit fish tanks around the studio wall so that I could watch tropical fish drift on by as I listened to lunatics for a living. They realised that I simply was not going to stay, no matter what, and finally let me be, although they did come back for a nibble or two over the next six months. Little did they know that it was the return of the anxiety attacks that were regrettably forcing me to make the decision to turn my back on something that was so good and so obviously successful.

After eventually getting 'clean' years later and being pill- and generally anxiety-free and looking back, it is one of my only life regrets that I was put in a situation where I had to give up something that I was really good at and enjoyed. I would never have left the job if fate hadn't dealt me this hand, but you can't be in a live talkback situation, out there on the high wire, delivering advice and consolation to the multitude, when your own head is spinning. So, I walked away.

6

Doctors and bad choices

It would be easy for you reading this to say that maybe I was allocating too much blame to a small white pill that I was taking each day, but by the time I left talkback radio, I'd been taking benzodiazepines for six years, and when I reflect back on who I was whilst taking them, compared to how I felt some years later when I'd kicked them and became free from anxiety and panic, I can clearly see some of the aberrant behavioural patterns and thoughts that went on in my life during those 13 years of addiction. (Google 'benzo-diazepine side effects' and you'll see what I'm referring to.)

One clear-cut thing that I did notice was my behaviour when drinking alcohol. Some of the weird things I'd do and say when boozed were not who I was but they manifested in the benzo days and stopped when I later got clean of the pre-scription drugs and that 'hole in my soul' was finally filled with happy living. Sadly, back then my life was one of constantly simmering, low-level anxiety every day from dawn to dusk due to the crippling monkey on my back.

I was now stranded in the middle of nothing and unemployed. Say goodbye to the talkback king.

In a short time, my relationship with the Princess also fell to pieces and I slipped through the cracks of my former life. I can assure you that it was a very unhappy period for me over the next few years, living on my own in a country cottage in sunny Hawke's Bay on the East Coast of New Zealand and working in the advertising sales part of the local radio station. I started having real problems with insomnia again and deep feelings of constant sadness. It was strange, because it wasn't depression; it was just this feeling of morbidity and a sense of hopelessness in everything I did. Anhedonia is apparently a term for those who can find no pleasure or joy out of anything, and that seemed to fit the bill perfectly. It wasn't that my exterior, material world was too bad. I was earning very good money in sales commissions at the radio station and taking trips to exotic places like Club Med in Tahiti, but deep down in my soul, I was very lost.

I'd started to read the occasional article which seemed to indicate that benzodiazepine tranquillisers were not a good look for long-term use, but I still hadn't given much thought to connecting the dots to the little white pills that I took daily and the way I constantly felt. The ultimate irony back then was that, in my naïve way of thinking, it was supposedly my taking of the Ativan that was the only thing that was preventing me from feeling psychologically worse than I did. Without the pills, I assumed, I would become a total psycho. How incredibly wrong that thinking was, as I'd find out.

One fine day, for some whimsical reason, I decided to delete the Ativan from my life, basically as they were just a hassle to keep getting from the doctor plus an emerging wish to kind of 'cleanse' myself from things that I perceived as having a modicum of control over me. I say this because at the same time I also decided that my pack-a-day cigarette habit also had to go. My approach to this shedding process was to not smoke until after 5pm (ridiculous) each day and, at the same time, very slowly shave a little bit off my daily regimen of benzo intake. Over the following months, I slowly whittled down the daily one milligram to halves at breakfast, early afternoon and before turning out the light at bedtime. I must reiterate again and again that it's extremely important that you follow a structured withdrawal plan when giving up a benzodiazepine addiction, because if you try to cut down too quickly you can go into epileptic fits, seizures and much worse. Over seven to eight months, I got it down from three pills to effectively one and a half pills a day, which was half the amount I'd taken over the previous eight years.

Once again, I'm sorry if all this detail sounds too specific for some of those reading my story, but this book is really being written to give help and hope to those millions, globally, who are still trapped in the vicious grip of tranquilliser addiction, so the details are very important. Incidentally, if you're wondering how many are addicted to benzos, right now in 2017, there are an officially estimated 2.3 million Britons in the UK alone who are hooked on prescription benzos, and that's just the tip of the global addiction iceberg. You can multiply that figure up dramatically for the number of addicts in the USA, and then there's rest of Europe and the Western world. Other recent research shows that anti-anxiety benzodiazepine drugs (yes, they're still being prescribed by the bucket load) accounted for nearly one-third of the 23,000 prescription drug overdoses in the US in 2013.

In this, my first attempt to quit, the gods must have been with me to a certain degree, as the process that I was following, albeit it was a bit rapid as it turned out, was fairly close to the recommended withdrawal procedure. Ironically, I found out much later that since I had not kept steadily increasing my daily dosage of 3mg of Ativan, like most addicts do chasing the full effect, and had remained constant throughout the 13 years, unbeknownst to me, I'd been experiencing what is known as ongoing daily, interdose withdrawals. Ativan is a fast-acting drug with a short 'half-life', which is the amount of time it takes for half the metabolites of the drug to leave the nervous system. By my not ramping up the dosage to match the tolerance my body had developed for Ativan over the previous years of intake, I was apparently going into mild withdrawal every single day, as the dose taken the previous day had worn off overnight. This explains a lot about my actions during those dark days and why every morning I woke up feeling full of fear, as if I had to start all over again doing the same climb up the same emotional mountain as the previous day, like a nasty version of *Groundhog Day* (if you've seen the movie, you'll know what I mean).

During this, my layman's attempt at withdrawal, I decided for some strange reason that the 'high' that the alcoholic drink Pernod and orange juice gave me would be my nightly substitute for the vanishing pills. Most evenings you could find me out on the verandah of my little cottage, watching the sun go down, puffing furiously on my after-5pm smokes and sipping on long glasses of iced, French aperitifs. Talk about deluded behaviour.

When I look back, I can see my whole uninformed approach of withdrawal was pretty laissez faire, which was probably why I soon found myself in a doctor's surgery complaining about my old nemesis of lack of sleep and sporadic feelings of high anxiety. Having got myself down to a smaller dose of the pills, I was obviously entering strong withdrawal reactions, which I didn't understand or recognise. Not giving the Ativan withdrawal the importance it deserved, I just figured that I was becoming more neurotic than usual. Chance is a fine thing because, as it turned out, I couldn't have chosen a worse doctor to go to (on the recommendation of a girlfriend). It wasn't until all hell broke loose in my life that I later found out the true back story on my newly chosen doctor.

Doctor Dan was a bit like another version of the famous Doctor Bob who tended to the Hollywood stars, including Elvis, prescribing a dazzling array of drugs to one and all without much question, but that was only a small part of Dr Dan's errant behaviour, which was to become obvious. There's actually a strange and perverse synchronicity about the choices of doctor that I made during the whole story of my addiction, because all of them actually worsened my situation and sped up my descent into an eventual nightmare.

My grandmother was an alternative thinker, being a member of the Fabian Society and a Christian Science believer. Their main line of thinking was that doctors were to be avoided at all cost and to leave healing to God, which is probably why she died at a young age of cancer, but this attitude also prevailed with my father, and we were bought up as children to view the GP fraternity as borderline charlatans. You would've thought I might have had better luck with my choices or even followed the family tradition and never gone near a doctor in the first place. How differently things would've turned out for me if I had. I should've known better, but again I was still in the grip of the 'white coat' syndrome, whereby you believe that the doctor knows best and went along with their diagnosis.

7

All hell broke loose

Don't ever wrestle with a pig. You'll both get dirty, but the pig will enjoy it.

When I explained my symptoms to a smiling and probably out of it Dr Dan, he asked the usual raft of odd questions and then gave me a prescription for 50mg twice daily of beta-blockers. This drug is usually given to high blood pressure sufferers, although they do have a short-term anxiety-reducing effect for situations like public speaking. I knew nothing about them but I took them and immediately my mind felt like a sledgehammer had hit me and my veins seemed like they'd turned to ice, which wasn't pleasant on top of the symptoms that I was already experiencing from my Ativan reduction. Terrible nightmares followed, along with diarrhoea and dizziness, so within days, I was back in his surgery complaining that I felt worse than before. He then did an inexcusable thing.

I had already told him that I'd worked hard that year to try to wean myself off a then eight-year tranquilliser habit, but he took little notice, instead telling me that I should try something different to help me sleep and, unbelievably, gave me Valium, which, of course, is part of the benzodiazepine group and the same drug cluster as Ativan. Because he'd called the Valium by its generic name of diazepam on the prescription, I assumed it was something new to help me overcome the curse of lack of sleep, because back then I really didn't know what I knew later about the different drugs, their names and dosages, etc., and the tenuous links between all of them. Once again, no explanation from a doctor of what was being prescribed. I dumped the beta-blockers and that night I took the diazepam (Valium) and my system went ballistic!

The gremlins in my psyche probably danced with joy at the arrival of more fresh benzos after months without any of the full regular dose feeding my nervous system since weaning myself down to a lower intake of Ativan. Within two days, I was on a real roller coaster of emotions and time slips. A cocktail of the previous beta-blockers, earlier withdrawal symptoms and now the Valium were all flying along at fast setting on the spin cycle in my brain and I was starting to fall into panicked confusion with absolutely no idea what was happening.

By this stage, it was approaching Christmas Day and the season to be jolly! People were packing up from work for the summer holidays. It was hot. Everyone was having fun and singing Christmas carols whilst I was feeling terrible, both physically and mentally, and not the slightest bit jolly. Profuse sweating, total sleeplessness and disorientation flooded my system, so again I traipsed back to Dr Dan but, by now, in a rather bad way. He started ranting that maybe I should try rebirthing, which is a regression process back to the womb and loved by the alternative thinkers (hippies). He rambled on about life and then said, 'This is what you need' and gave me another prescription telling me to bin the Valium and Ativan combo that I had been taking. Dangerous times were now approaching.

I have no trouble in recounting this as it is deeply etched in my mind as surely as it would've been if someone had slipped me an LSD 'acid' trip without my knowledge. It was a beautiful summer's evening when I again left his surgery and went to the 24-hour pharmacy to get my script filled. When the pharmacist handed the drugs over to me he asked if I was fully aware of what I was taking and inquired as to whether Dr Dan had given me any information. He seemed to be taking a special interest in what he was giving me, as he had made a point of coming around from behind his work station and out into the pharmacy to talk with me. This should've rung warning bells, but I just nodded in my spaced-out view of what was going on. His parting instructions were 'Well, whatever you do, don't suddenly stop taking this medication, as you will experience some quite serious problems.' It didn't really register with me, as I figured that this was standard practice, so I didn't absorb the implications of what he was saying.

So, childlike, I again did as I was told by Dr Dan and the pharmacist and went home to take my new drugs without any idea as to what they were for, strength of dose or any knowledge of potential side effects. Given what I know now, I find it very hard to believe that I could be so naïve, but how many of you reading this book would've actually questioned your doctor or pharmacist when you were first prescribed tranquillisers? Very few, I would think.

It was now four days before Christmas Day. That night, I swallowed the first round of capsules that Dr Dan had prescribed to me and what ensued borders on the criminal. By the early hours of the following morning, I was wide awake, panic-stricken, with a dry mouth like the bottom of a birdcage and having the most horrific thought patterns that would make *Game of Thrones* look like a walk in the park. I find it hard now to specifically describe what it was like, as it was such a whirlwind ride of mood swings and pan-icked emotions, but I can clearly remember feeling as if I'd left my body and was only a fraction away from going com-pletely out of control. Fortunately, my work obligations had finished for the summer, as I couldn't have gone to work.

I stayed indoors all the next day in a state of high distress and hot as hell from the summer sun beating down on the cottage, but by that night, as darkness descended, things were really getting dangerous to the degree that I thought I was heading past the tipping point and close to going insane or out of control. One weird thing that I can remember doing was that every few hours I would get in my car and drive around the block just to maintain a sense of familiar surroundings, but I was rapidly losing touch with any reality and red-line was approaching.

I rang Dr Dan the following day in a jabbering, sleep-deprived panic and told him what was happening and his response was that he'd done as much as he could to help me and anyway he was going away for his Christmas vacation and hung up the phone. Unbelievable, really! I tried ringing a couple of other random doctors from the phone book but, as you can imagine, no doctor upon hearing from a gabbling stranger about pills and hallucinatory reactions is going to get involved in another doctor's business, so I got no joy there.

It was only when I rang a good friend of mine who had been a nurse in Vietnam and had risen to be the Matron at a private hospital that things started to be pulled back into line. She came over to my home, took one look at me and the pills I was taking and commandeered the situation.

We located another doctor who saw me immediately and told me that the drugs I had been prescribed by Dr Dan were a heavy drug called Ascendin and also an antidepressant known as Prothiaden. This double dosage was bad enough, but the reason why I was spinning out so badly was because the milligram dose Dr Dan had given me was, believe it or not, apparently *10 times* above the accepted medical guide-lines' maximum dose and would only be prescribed in extreme circumstances, such as someone going berserk or self-harming whilst locked in a psychiatric unit. To think this all started because I simply wanted a decent night's sleep!

8

———

Upon reflection

The new doctor we'd located gradually took me down off the frenzied drug plateau I was on (Happy Christmas, Rob), and when I told him about coming off the benzos and the cigarettes throughout the previous year he simply said that it would be easier if I went back to square one and lit up a smoke and took half an Ativan and went to bed. Only those with an addiction to drugs, cigarettes or alcohol, etc. can know that infantile sense of relief and perverse pleasure of abrogation of responsibility when an authority like a doctor has given you that sort of permission, even though it was completely counterproductive to what I'd tried to achieve over the last year. Deep down, we're all children and although it's totally pathetic, when doctor says do this or that, sometimes if you're 'under the gun' as I was at that point, it's just plain nice to be given an excuse to do what the doctor instructs, so I sat round for the next few days chilled on a pill and chain smoking.

When I'd calmed down to a modicum of sanity, it was the beginning of the New Year. I'd started to plot what to do about Dr Dan. However, the local law enforcement officers took care of that problem when they coincidentally raided his house whilst he was still away on his holiday break and allegedly found a stack of cannabis plants growing hydroponically in his ceiling.

Although I've never ascertained the truth of the matter, I am led to believe that the other doctor who had saved me from potential madness by getting me down out of my 'tree', apparently laid a complaint to the New Zealand Medical Council about the overdosing of the drug that Dr Dan had given me and the upshot was that Dan, as I understand it, was put on a limited prescribing list and had restrictions put on his practice.

I guess it was all part of my karmic learning curve that Dr Dan and my paths had crossed and that I had ended up letting him use me as a pharmaceutical dartboard, but it was only a portent of the future and what was still awaiting me. This was just the start of the real trip to the edge of my sanity!

Oh, no, readers … this episode was nothing compared to what was to come. Yes, indeed, much worse was waiting for me in the not-too-distant future. In fact, it would be fair to say that it would take another five years, until 1993, before I emerged out of my detox nightmare, completely clean and, like a newborn foal, shaky on my feet, but pill free!

It's probably worthwhile to stop here for a breather and have an overview of the whole withdrawal process before we plough on with my story. Unfortunately, being free of the pharmaceuticals running through your nervous system is only the beginning of the cleansing process. From the long tail of emotional wreckage, known as your former addicted life, the task in hand is to then put yourself back together and that's the hard bit. It's rather like deciding to stop taking the pills and then standing still on the train track of all you've ever known yourself to be, whilst the past 13 years, in fact, all your life's experiences, run straight over the top of you like a speeding train, breaking you into a million small fragments. Then the challenge is to reassemble yourself as a shiny, new person, minus any past or drug-induced influences. A tall order you may say, but I'm here to tell you it can be done. And I can guarantee you that this saga of mine does have a positive and happy outcome, making all the trials and tribulations worthwhile.

Think about that. Imagine it! Freedom from those chemical shackles that have been dragging along behind you like a slushing pile of wet rope for all those past years of your half-lived life. Yes, you can turn around and cut that wet rope entangled on your soul and feel it slowly drop away from your very being. I say that because I think it's important that I strongly emphasise that it really is worth it to free yourself of addiction of any kind, before plunging you into what comes next in my story. I want to encourage you to do what I did and take the life-altering decision to escape from benzodiazepines and similar prescription drugs.

However, I don't want you to be frightened off by what happened to me, as that would be counterproductive to the whole reason for my writing this book. The truth is that everything unfortunate that occurred in my life, which, at times, threatened my very existence, ended up being the absolutely best things in the long run.

We only see a small portion of the big picture of our life at the time that we live it, and we act like that's the ongoing reality, when it's not. We must trust the process and believe in the bigger picture. As I've indicated, I will point you to forums and links that will guarantee that you don't need to go it alone like I did. Also, it's important to point out that there is no hard fast template that says the exact same things that happened to me will happen to anyone giving up prescription benzo drugs. There is no one-size-fits-all experience common to everyone going into recovery and you may be one of the lucky ones that breezes through withdrawal, but for most of those addicted to benzos, there is certainly a lot of symptomatic commonality in the withdrawal process and eventual recovery.

9

The 'shrink'

From my Dr Dan experience onwards, the next five years of my life is the real nub of this book, and the experiences I encountered are often like some horror movie. But it's a story that needs to be told if only for my redemption and the lessons learnt that I need to pass on to you.

Apparently, benzos have the capacity to interfere with your episodic memory, while leaving the semantic memory relatively intact, but I don't think I have any memory retention issues about those days. Semantic memory is the recollection of generalised information about the world, untied to the specific events that occurred as the knowledge was encoded in your mind. Episodic memory is the ability to recall one's personal experience of actual events. Benzodiazepines can significantly disrupt the memory of such events, which would explain their use as 'date rape' drugs.

Everything that happened to me, though, is burnt so

episodically into my memory hard drive that even years later I'm having no problems going back, as every minute detail flows onto my keyboard and into this book. I have, however, found it stressful and personally upsetting to go back and tell my story, but it must be done.

After the Dr Dan experience, the summer break had finished and I tried to get back to my work at the radio station, but I was so frazzled mentally that within weeks, I resigned from my job and lapsed into a vacuum of hopelessness.

By now I was understandably gun-shy from my experiences with the mainstream medical fraternity, so I had a small flirtation with the alternative sector and consulted an anthroposophical doctor, who followed the teachings of 20th-century philosopher and occultist Rudolf Steiner. Although the doctor was well-intentioned, his diagnosis was that my sleeplessness and anxiety symptoms were largely caused by Ahriman (their version of the devil) entering my liver at night, so his advice was for me to get up at 3am each morning and take some drops he'd prescribed and this would cleanse my liver, sort me out and get rid of Ahriman all at once.

Given sleep was my big issue, having to set my alarm to wake up from a half-slumber and take a potion to help me sleep seemed to conflict with the whole reason for trying to stay asleep, so I flagged that alternative concept away.

Bear in mind that I was now back where I was a year earlier and again taking my daily round of Ativan. They say that 'what doesn't kill you makes you stronger', but sometimes the whole point of going on can seem hopeless. Fortunately, I appear to have been blessed with a very strong will, which was to stand me in good stead over the coming traumatic years.

I now found that living in my little cottage in Hawke's Bay had become tainted with the memories of my summer experience of borderline madness. Disenchantment with my life in general had set in, so I decided to return to where I perceived the world as being that of happier times. I packed up and headed back to sunny Queensland, Australia, and Surfers Paradise on the eastern Gold Coast. I'd lived there before and the thought of the sound of the sea and constant warmth from the sun seemed to have a womb-like appeal to me and would, hopefully, offer a mental antidote for my last 10 years in New Zealand.

I flew out of New Zealand to Brisbane and then moved into a condo on the main beach at Surfers Paradise, which was only designed for tourists short term and didn't have a kitchen, so I usually started my day sitting on the end of my bed in my tenth-storey burrow, gazing out at morning paradise with the 'shaving foam' waves rolling in, munching on my daily bowl of cornflakes, bananas and milk as I prepared to head off to work at my new job as a media sales rep on the Gold Coast.

Under normal circumstances it would've been the perfect job. The radio station that I'd started working for was located only about an hour up the freeway in Brisbane City. They provided me with a serviced office on the ninth floor of an ultra-modern steel and glass tower block and the freedom to do whatever I wanted as long as I produced results.

The sun was always shining and long, expense-account client lunches were the order of the day as I went about conjuring up great sales results, but here I was again, laughing on the outside but very sad deep down in my heart and my anxious little soul (and still popping my daily Ativan).

I felt constant hopelessness as to ever getting my life back on track after the failure in New Zealand to go any further forward in tidying up my life. After all the drama I'd been through, nothing had changed. I was still taking the benzos and as dependent on them as ever and still totally unaware of the caustic effect they were having on my very being.

By chance, I read a front-cover story in *Time* magazine about depression and anxiety, etc. and was struck by a line that talked about feelings of 'constant sadness' as opposed to feeling depressed. This resonated with me and how I felt so, still ignorant of the actual cause being the pills, I decided to see what could be done about it and, hopefully, make an all-out effort once again to rectify things.

Returning to my naïve default position of trusting general practitioners, I spoke to the Gold Coast doctor who was now prescribing my Ativan and asked him to arrange for a complete physical check-up.

If that came up as normal then I wanted him to recommend a psychologist for my 'constant emotional sadness', which is exactly how it played out as all the tests, from barium meals for my insides to bloods to X-rays, all came back healthy and clear.

Up until this point in my life, I'd always surfed along the tops of my feelings and followed the mainstream medical bouncing ball, albeit with some bad results, but I'd never walked through the door into exploring the deeper machinations of my troubled soul, so it was a new experience for me to consult with a 'shrink'.

The person my Gold Coast doctor sent me to was a very

interesting and complex character and, as it turned out, was not a psychologist but a psychiatrist. For the uninitiated, the difference is that only psychiatrists are medically trained practitioners and can therefore prescribe drugs, which again in hindsight was an initial plus but eventually a very big negative as things transpired.

He was English and had practised in New Zealand, but the probable attraction of consulting him was that he also had had media experience, so given my radio background, we immediately had mutually good connections and a jumping-off point to get inside my head.

It's an interesting experience going into analysis, as most Americans would testify. (You're not on the bus in the States unless you have a therapist.) Doctor Zed was good at his craft and explained quite lot of the inner workings of the subconscious and unconscious mind to me but, fascinating though it was, it really didn't alter the fact that, despite discussing my dependency with him, I was still addicted to Ativan, which he was now also prescribing to me.

Like, what was I doing there if that was the case? It occurred to me that it was a bit like an alcoholic spending an hour in analysis, paying A$120 for the privilege and then being given a bottle of booze on the way out!

Fortunately, the Australian Medicare system allowed me to claim a large part of the hourly fee, so I spent many sessions with Dr Zed and I must be honest that at that juncture, I think it was beneficial to me, if for no other reason than it allowed me for the first time in my life to pour out my heart and soul about my childhood, a failed marriage, emotional loss and anxiety freak-outs.

Apparently, there is a psychological paradox that when

you talk about something you've never discussed with any-one, the mere manifesting of those inner demons into the verbal 'open air' causes the internal pain of the mind to evaporate them to quite a large degree. I think the Catholic Church cornered the franchise on that one with the concept of the confessional box back in the Dark Ages.

Eventually, the Brisbane-based radio station promoted me up from Surfers Paradise on the Gold Coast to their head office. Living back in the city where I'd married my wife nearly 18 years earlier and the associated memories was a quirky experience, but I went with it and floated along in a sort of psychic hold pattern. I'd hooked up with a nightclub-bing bunch of friends, so the weekends were spent around the city drinking, out of it on smoke and basically just repeating the past, only this time I was now older and chem-ically dependent on Ativan.

The drug Ecstasy was big on the scene back then but I never tried it, as I heard the fallout the next day sounded like something that I was contending with anyway. Why would I want to pay money for another drug that would make me even more anxious and out of balance than I already was? There are many interesting anecdotes about that particular time of my life in Brisbane City that I could tell you, but the purpose of this book is to take you through my experiences of giving up prescription drugs and shedding my depen-dency on Ativan, so we'll just have to save that for the movie.

Life took on a different hue when I met a gorgeous young 'English rose' who was visiting her sister in Brisbane and, to cut a long story short, she showed me a lot of good rea-sons why I should follow her back to England for more of her kinky ways! I'd always liked women younger than myself, which is not unusual, and she had 'daddy issues', so we were a perfect fit for mutually assured destruction, otherwise known as MAD — very appropriate.

Meanwhile, since moving up from the Gold Coast, I'd continued seeing Dr Zed each week in his Brisbane offices but still with no further focus on the question of my Ativan dependence being discussed at our consultations. He must've known from experience that a bonfire would be lit if I'd tried to give up the benzos and maybe he just thought he was sparing me the greater of two evils.

It had now got to the point where our meetings were more like a catch-up between a couple of blokes at the hotel yarning over the events of the day. The process of transference sets you up for that and it probably would've gone on for ages if I hadn't met Decca, my new-found English, female addiction. The only problem was that one of the side effects of benzos is that they can tangle with your libido, so it was often a game of sexual Russian roulette as to how a romp in the sack would turn out!

10

London calling

During my time in Australia, I'd taken out Australian citizenship without having to relinquish my New Zealand status, which gave me two passports.

My grandmother was from Edinburgh in Scotland, giving me the automatic right to an English work permit, so after spending quite a bit of bureaucratic time getting things sorted, I jetted out of Brisbane bound for London and the arms of sweet Decca, who had since returned to the UK.

I had purposely waited till May to migrate, as that was the usual start of the English summer, but it was to turn out to be a waste of time as the 'summer' that I flew into was so interminably cold and wet that the Brits had to cancel one complete weekend of the traditional Wimbledon tennis tournament, for the first time in 113 years.

Cold and miserable, fish-grey English days surrounded me, with daylight not fully formed until around 10.30 am and then what watery sun that did appear would go down again in the late afternoon and turn into premature night-time. (Easy to see why the Brits invented sado-masochism and depression with weather like that to contend with. It's enough to make anyone feel depressed.)

Prior to leaving Australia, I had sourced a list of introductions to 10 of the top radio executives in London and around the UK, which had been supplied to me by influential radio people both in Australia and New Zealand, so I thought I was locked and loaded for a bright, new future.

I also had a medical letter and a month's ongoing prescription for Ativan, courtesy of Dr Zed, clutched in my hot little hand. Other than the rubbish weather, what could go wrong?

Plenty. That's what!

I don't know whether you've ever experienced those times when, despite all your best efforts, destiny seems to grab you by the throat and spin you around until all your plans fly to pieces and the world starts to go out of control. Well, that's exactly what happened as soon as I landed in London from Australia. The plan was to stay with a close relative who had invited me to come over and stay until I got locked into the London work scene and found good accommodation. I'd communicated many times with her before leaving Australia with no inkling of what she was really like but, unfortunately, she turned out, upon arrival, to be the bitch from hell.

She had a place not far out of central London at Clapham Junction in the southwest area near Lavender Hill, which was set in a row of houses all connected like sardines in a can, like what you'd see on TV's *Coronation Street* (popular programme but not shown in US).

I'd flown all day and night from Australia, so was naturally dog-tired after around 28 hours' flying time, but when I arrived by taxi to her place there was no one there to meet me so I had to sit out on the pavement on my suitcases in the freezing cold for most of the day until said charitable relative finally got home from work in the city.

What was meant to be a promised bed for me to sleep on turned out to be on the floor and on top of that, she was clearly not a very nice person.

On the second week, my father in New Zealand died, I had my briefcase stolen, Decca, the English rose, had gone back to her wealthy stockbroker boyfriend out in Buckinghamshire, and so the unravelling of yours truly continued at a relentless pace.

My bank in London, NatWest, temporarily lost all record of my bank account, the Yanks were invading Iraq for the first Gulf War, and the UK was gripped in a bad Thatcherite recession. Talk about good timing. If I didn't need tranquillisers before, I certainly did then.

By now you'll be getting the picture that the stress was starting to really pile up. To top it off, I came down with a very bad dose of influenza whilst the relative from hell continued to torment me till I finally fled to the apartment upstairs, owned by a paranoid schizophrenic whose wealthy father paid him a large allowance to stay away from the family.

His main attraction was that he loathed my relative living below him, so he was only too pleased to give me a broken-down old bedroom in his flat, if only to piss her off. I spent most of my nights with a knife jammed in the bedroom door because my new-found chum, Mark, laboured under the delusion that he had murdered someone on a trip to the home of the devil, New Orleans (which he may well have), so I would hear him prowling around at night, high as a kite, muttering to himself about psychotic death and violence somewhere in the heart of America.

This may all sound like a bit of a challenge, but destiny was yet to play her finest hand and emphatically force the beginning of my long journey to eventual freedom from Ativan.

At the time, what came next didn't look like any sort of a plus, but that's how life often works when you look back and see the hidden silver lining in what seemed on the surface to be like a terrible part of your life.

11

Prescription reality check in Clapham

I was starting to run out of Ativan but was not overly concerned as I had a prescription and a letter from Doctor Zed in Australia, so I booked an appointment with a local doctor in Clapham Junction with the intention of loading up on another month's supply of pills and life would go on as I sought to lock onto living in London and into the radio bigtime.

I should mention that the bigger picture was to get established in media, travel regularly to Europe, etc. and live in England permanently.

But that all changed when I sat down in front of an earnest-looking, little Indian doctor and he spelt out the reality of my situation in no uncertain terms.

It turned out that, unbeknownst to me, there were massive class-action litigations going on through the English courts by those addicted to benzodiazepines against the huge drug companies who manufactured most of the benzo group of drugs globally, including Ativan.

In the 1980s, 17,000 claimants began a class action against the pharmaceutical manufacturers Roche Products and John Wyeth, and this had spooked doctors up and down the United Kingdom. Unfortunately, procedural delays, technical motions and escalating costs eventually prevented the cases actually coming to trial. A small group attempted to continue unrepresented as litigants in person, but failed. The manufacturers' total legal costs, £35 million, were awarded but not enforced against one of those final litigants, a Mr Michael Behan, who was last heard of working for a local British MP.

There were calls for inquiries from the House of Lords in the British Parliament and the legal aid bills for those addicted claimants were going through the roof (this aid was eventually stopped due to skyrocketing costs to the British Government). and slowly, it all faded away, being filed in the too-hard basket, and that was the situation I had unwittingly landed into in the UK in the early nineties.

Until I met that Indian doctor on that fateful morning in downtown Clapham, I'd long ago stuffed the memory into the back of my mind of my horrific experience with Dr Dan back in New Zealand a few years earlier and simply saw my daily input of Ativan as just a fact of my everyday life that I would have to contend with. You know how it goes. You realise it's something that you should address, like giving up smoking, but you never seem to get around to it. Like, is there ever a perfect day to give up anything addictive? You also forget about how much better you used to feel all those years back when you weren't reliant on a chemical crutch to get through your day.

However, on that day in Clapham Junction, all roads in my life collided into one nasty realisation.

The Indian doctor explained to me that in the UK most doctors were now trying to cut back on prescribing benzos for fear of being sued for medical misadventure. Only in certain cases, such as death or grief situations, were they still giving them out, and that the British Government had instructed the medical profession to begin cutting down the benzo intake of their existing patients on a national basis.

So here I was, trying to get more when less was the message. He must've seen the panicked look on my face because he agreed to give me a script for another 30-day's supply of Ativan, but told me that I wouldn't be getting any more and to try other doctors would be a waste of time, as I was now registered in the National Health database.

I've always been very aware of the synchronicity of omens and events in the way I've conducted my life, so when I wandered out of that clinic in Clapham, I knew the cosmic tectonic plates in my world had shifted, and not in a good way. I filled my Ativan script and scuttled back to my temporary lodgings at 'Camp Schizo' to find my new-found flatmate smashed on some evil concoction, so it became clear to me that it was time to move on. I had to find an alternative to staying there, but where? I was a stranger in a strange land.

How could my dreams of living in England, working on the radio and travelling the continent with sexy Decca have gone so horribly wrong? And now to top it off, my previous conveniently ignored addiction had suddenly become a very scary reality. I knew the game was over for Mr Rob and his big migration plans, but what to do?

I still had most of my belongings stored out at Heathrow Airport on the edge of Greater London at a cost of 70 quid a day, the polite rejection letters were starting to trickle back from various radio stations that I had sent my résumé to, and all my forays around downtown London were sucking up what money I still had in the bank (yes, they had found it again).

Feeling anxious and depressed, I caught a train from Paddington Station in central London and fled south to the beautiful Cornwall coast where some of my ancestors had apparently lived. Cooped up in a little bedsit run by two kindly lesbians in Padstow, somewhere near Bodmin on the southern English coast, riddled with flu and lost as lost can be, I finally succumbed to it all and crashed out, sleeping for about three days.

When the energy returned, I briefly roamed around places nearby, like Tintagel, where Merlin was supposedly born according to the Arthurian legends of Camelot, and the nearby lake near Bodmin where the hand of the Lady of the Lake apparently emerged from the water, clutching the sword Excalibur.

After about a week, I returned to London leaving the flowering fields of Cornwall's pink frith and yellow rape behind me for the first and last time.

Disembarking from the train back in London, I was walking dejectedly through the famous Aussie and Kiwi expat area of Earls Court. It was blowing a gale; sleet was stinging my face. My umbrella gave up battling the elements, inverting inside out.

'Bugger this,' I thought. 'It's over.'

Time to be like a good general and retreat back to base and regroup in Australia again where the sun shone and prescriptions for my meds were easy to get. I'd tried to conquer England and failed. No one's perfect!

At the same time, I looked across the street and there, on a travel agency window, emblazoned in large letters, were the words 'British Airways, one-way flight to Australia, only £379 — great value'. It was like a synchronistic omen. That was it! I'd been beaten down and the ultimate kicker was I was now also an aware addict, cast adrift with no legal supplier. Survival time had arrived! Towing my suitcase behind me, I stumbled into the travel agency and asked a young agent to book me on the advertised flight back to Sydney, Australia.

I was so pissed off about my life in general that I told him to arrange for a stop-off in Bangkok so I could lose my miserable self in the bars of the 'heart of darkness' in sleazy old Thailand, but even that was not meant to be. He tried to book me hotel accommodation and a flight into Bangkok from London and then drily informed me that the *whole* of Thailand was booked out, which he and I both knew was an impossibility. Apparently, as my luck would have it, across that week the magnetic field around the planet had been bombarded by sun flare radiation that was so dramatically intense and close to the Earth, that even the French Concorde jet was flying at low levels (bear in mind, this was the nineties) and globally the primitive computer networks of the day were consequently going haywire.

Everything was a blur from there onwards until a few days later, I touched down around midnight in Sydney, Australia, after another gruelling 28-hour flight jammed up in cattle class with smelly, sweating Brits heading to the sunny beaches of Bondi or similar.

I'd only lasted in England for about four months, so when I got back to Sydney it was still winter. A friend of mine from my radio days met me at the airport with the greeting 'Mate, what's happened? You look like a ghost', which I did. I'd lost a huge amount of weight from the stress of the English experience and I was not a happy boy, but I knew my first priority was to sort out my next prescription of Ativan. Nothing like a dependency to get you focused. They say if you want to know if you're addicted to something, just stop taking it and you'll find out, but I didn't need to play that game; I knew that I was in trouble. The next day, I was on the phone to Dr Zed, my shrink in Queensland, and he obligingly couriered me down a prescription, which took the urgency out of things for the moment.

I was sleeping on the floor (again) at my mate's place in Sydney in a freezing atrium on an airbed that slowly deflated overnight, so within a few days I'd had enough. I bought myself a late-model Ford Falcon and drove about 10 hours north and back to the inner sanctum of my good friends Frank and Ava, who owned a very cool and funky house perched right on the ocean at a place called South Golden Beach, just north of the alternative hippie capital of Australia, Byron Bay.

Whilst living in Brisbane and prior to taking off on my disastrous trip to the UK, I had spent many wild days and nights at the beach house with Frank and his other half, the ebullient Ava, and their eclectic bunch of friends.

They both worked over the Queensland state border in

Brisbane and used to commute north for the week and then return home for the weekend, which would be spent in full-throttle partying with friends from north, south, east and west pouring in for a couple of days of good times. And they were exceptionally good times, with long nights lolling in the outdoor spa pool, sucking up champagne under the starry Australian skies.

Upon my arrival up from Sydney, I stayed with them for a few days until I got my breath back and then headed north over the border to Brisbane in a very despondent state of mind. My overseas trip was meant to have been my finest hour and it had turned out to be my biggest bloody failure.

Again, in hindsight, I came to view the whole English experience as a blessing, because if I hadn't gone there, failed and been confronted with the harsh reality of my pill addiction and been given the beginning of correct information on the truth about benzos, I may still be in the land of misery.

Blessings can often come in very strange disguises.

I've always had the resilience to pick myself up and get back into what needed to be done, so I soon found myself an apartment in Brisbane and started calling up friends and thinking about work, as by this time I was nearly broke.

There you have it pretty much in a nutshell. So here endeth the back story of my younger life and how I ended up addicted to prescription drugs.

12

Fleeing back to Australia

Into Hell we go ...

From here on, it is all about the madness and the savage dogs of hell that are cut loose when you decide to stop taking the benzodiazepines.

Up to this point, the events I've written about have really been to give you an overview of my life and personality in the hope that you may find some connection to your own life story, particularly if you're caught up in the same benzo dependency trap.

I'm working on the principle that most people reading this book will be trying to find a map of courage to help them take that first step towards settling that mortgage on their own soul, namely by dumping their benzos or Zops (sleeping tablets).

Yes, for the first time I'm throwing sleepers like the Z's, as they're known, into the mix.

Sleeping tablets, like Zopiclone, are mainly of a similar group to benzodiazepines (non-benzo hypnotics, to be precise) and are now as big a problem as the anxiolytic benzos like Ativan, Valium or Xanax. So, don't be fooled into thinking that your nightly dose of Zopiclone is anything less than potentially addictive if used for more than 2-6 weeks and can be extremely hard to withdraw from. Zopiclone is a tricky drug, as it does work in giving you what seems like 'sleep' but, essentially, you're drugged and are getting the so-called sleep due to its anti-anxiety effects, not normal REM sleep, which is where your brain washes away the rubbish of the temporary files from your previous day's activities.

If you're taking Ambien or pills similar to Zopiclone, you may notice that when you awake from maybe nine hours' slumber, you still don't feel truly rested or any less stressed.

The one area where they do have a practical use, in my opinion, is if you're travelling overseas on a long-haul flight and you want to try to get some chill time and also when you land in a foreign country and you're jet-lagged, then half a Zopiclone will help you get some shuteye even if it is only to turn off your thinking for a while.

As a sidebar regarding sleep, it pays to not panic when you wake in the wee small hours of the morning after only around four hours of normal sleep, as this is what's meant to naturally happen. Prior to the invention of the electric light and our crazed modern world, people invariably went to bed as soon as it got dark, which meant they woke up in the middle of the night after only about four hours in bed. In pre-light-bulb days, it was quite normal for people to then get up, visit a neighbour, drink tea or have sex over the next hour or so and eventually go back to bed and happily fall asleep for another four hours, giving them the usual eight hours' sleep. I used to stress out when I woke after only a few hours' sleep but since discovering that it's quite normal, I just relax and do some deep breathing or maybe check outside and then just drift back to sleep. The key to it is to accept it as normal to wake up after around 4 hours and not get your panties in a bunch about it!

Now, it's time to get back down to the business of ridding myself of the accursed benzos!

After my disastrous trip to England, I had now gone full circle and was once again back living in Brisbane, Australia. It'd only been five or six months since leaving there for the UK, with just a lot of hardship and only an empty wallet to show for it.

The internet was generally available back then, but technology was still only in pre-broadband, dial-up mode and mainly found in offices or home computers for geeks. I had virtually nil tech experience so researching how to go about the task in hand of giving up benzo dependency required physically finding various self-help people or government agencies that specialised in alcohol or drug addiction.

If it was nowadays, by accessing the 'net', I could've breezed through many online sites which were offering advice and case studies, but nothing like that was available to me at the time, so I had to foot slog it around the city in search of help and information.

TRANX, which is an Australasian addiction network now known as Reconnexion (http://www.reconnexion.org.au), was my first port of call, but the only help I got from them was a pile of very official-looking books on the withdrawal process and what to expect. When I read through the material as to what could potentially happen, I considered forgetting the whole idea, as some of the side effects of withdrawal listed by TRANX were horrific, but they turned out to be correct.

They gave me an appointment with a woman who was obviously new to the counselling field, as she managed to treat me like a low-life addict within five minutes of our first conversation. I told her that not all addicts were liars (although most heavy drug users usually are) and moved on, clutching my pile of well-meaning brochures.

It's probably worthwhile now to draw the wide distinction between prescription pill users and the underworld of the heavy drugs like heroin, P, meth, coke, etc. You never hear of a bunch of housewives or pill people, like myself, getting together to have benzo parties, but in the scene of recreational hard drugs that's exactly what they're taken for. Shot up with the needle, snorted, whatever. The whole idea for the meth 'tweakers' and dope fiends is to party and get out of it, but not so for the poor ol' benzo users.

The pill addict is a totally different breed of animal to the dope freaks, which is quite an important distinction. The reason I say that is that many prescription drug addicts, such as I was, end up there by medical misadventure and through no fault of their own. A doctor had prescribed them a drug with the assurance that it would be good for a specific presented symptom, without ever detailing the pitfalls, so the onus of blame lies with the doctor, not the patient, in my estimation.

The interesting thing is that people who were prescribed

tranquillisers for non-anxiety reasons still ended up exhibiting all the same anxiety-driven, nightmare side effects and withdrawal symptoms as those who had been prescribed benzos for anxiety, which clearly points to the nature of these drugs, regardless of why you started taking them in the first place.

No fear, no favour, has the bitch goddess of benzo!

It's also important to point out that people who are addicted to these drugs nearly always feel a sense of shame or guilt, as if it was somehow their fault and that they were weak because they had ended up in an addicted predicament.

I know in my case that was exactly how I felt and even now I'm hesitant about publishing this book because I mistakenly still feel that I will be perceived as weak for ever having taken the pills. And, hey, everyone knows only weak people take pills? Yeah, right! Get over that one. Get a firm mental fix on the fact that it's not your fault. It's the fault of the medical professionals that prescribed them to you for not clearly explaining the potential pitfalls, not yours. Benzodiazepine dependency is nothing to be ashamed of. It is not a matter of an addictive personality but of a pharmacological insult put upon you, for which you're not to blame. The only difference between a drug addict and the rest of society is the drug.

Whilst scouting around for reliable research on tranquillisers I still managed to get it together and form my own business, marketing print advertising in Queensland.

I got it up and running to the point where I was getting steady client appointments and then I decided that all the wandering around trying to find advice about self-detoxing from Ativan was fruitless. The time had come to put on my big-boy's pants and start the process of cutting down my daily pill intake and take the plunge into the unknown world of withdrawal.

Yes, the day of reckoning had arrived, and based on my overseas experience in London and everything else that had held me captive in the past, I knew there was to be no going back. The pills had to go. I had to be free to live my life without any artificial crutch, especially one that was causing, not solving, the anxiety issues.

The process of withdrawal and detox is definitely not to be taken lightly. None of this 'I think I'll just stop taking these pills' attitude.

If you've been addicted for a protracted period of time, sudden withdrawal (cold turkey) can bring on any of these: epileptic, grand mal seizure fits, suicide, cardiac arrest, hallucinations, heart attacks and strokes.

That road leads to madness. Don't do it. Leave it for the turkeys at Christmas.

The basic premise of withdrawal, or tapering, as some people prefer to call it, is that you gradually cut down by shaving a small fraction off your daily intake over many weeks.

Based on the information in the books TRANX had given me, I knew from the withdrawal symptoms they had charted that I could expect to experience at the very least:

- extreme anxiety

- restlessness

- irritability

- insomnia

- headaches

- poor concentration

- depression

- depersonalisation

- panic attacks

- sweating

- racing heart

- muscle tension

- tightness in the chest

- difficulty breathing

- tremor

- nausea, vomiting, or diarrhoea

- agoraphobia (fear of open spaces and crowds)

- loss of memory

- rapid mood changes

- shaking inwardly and outwardly

- loss of balance

- flu-like symptoms

- abdominal pain and cramps

- feelings of the ground moving

People who go into rehabilitation to get over alcohol or opiate addictions, such as Oxycontin or Vicodin, initially struggle with rebound anxiety, insomnia and some of the symptoms listed above, but such problems subside in a relatively short period of time, often in a matter of mere weeks, after completing the discontinuation process.

But not so with the benzos!

The down-regulation of GABA mediation of nerve cells is the single defining problem that differentiates benzodiazepine recovery from that of any other substance such as heroin, etc.

With this in mind, it would be far more accurate to say that people who are dependent on benzodiazepines are not so much addicted to the benzo itself but to GABA. and their suffering in tapering withdrawal is a result of the ceasing of a continual daily benzodiazepine GABA intake. The body's *natural* GABA neurotransmitter, which benzodiazepine pills have caused to be unavailable in sufficient amount due to you providing a chemical GABA substitute over the years, has caused the brain to long ago give up the natural manufacturing of GABA in favour of the benzo substitute.

When you go into self-detox and start tapering, you stop supplying the brain with enough artificial GABA, via the daily benzo, and the brain is still not producing any natural GABA and without enough GABA, neurons in the brain then start to fire too often and too easily causing the resulting high anxiety, so now you're in no-man's-land ... but not for ever, as the brain gradually starts the engines and begins producing real brain GABA, and that is the beginning of your doorway to eventual peace and freedom.

But this is all academic and not much use to you in the real world until you make the big decision to give it a go and start the serious procedure of giving up benzos...

PART II

Waltzing with the Devil, Narcotics Anonymous and Withdrawal

13

In off the deep end

The summers in Brisbane are very hot with regular daily temperatures in the mid-30s Celsius with extremely high humidity, so going into withdrawal in those conditions didn't help, although I guess it was probably better than being in cold, bleak, depressing winter days.

I say this because once I entered phase two, emotional withdrawal, a few months further down the track, post physical self-detox, the emotional detox was actually the worse of the two, with waves of blinding, reactive depression becoming all-encompassing like dark angels of doom, so the gloomy shades of winter don't help your mood. Better to start to detox when it's warm, if possible.

Came a hot Friday around about mid-January 1992 when I leapt in off the deep end of my life and started a programme of slowly shaving portions off the pills I was taking.

A fraction shaved off a small pill may sound infinitesimal,

but unless you understand how the milligrams of different benzos work, it must be clearly understood that just a fraction shaved off a 1mg pill, or even a half pill, can have huge effects on your nervous system and chemically dependent mental and physical state.

From everything I had read, I figured the trick was to shave the fractions off the morning dose for a week or two, take a week's break and then do the same thing the next week off the remaining pills I was taking, until I was down to (shudder) zero. (Turns out later that I should've started on the night-time dose but, if you'll excuse the pun, I was flying in the dark back then.)

You can't imagine how scary this all seemed to me after 13 years of having my daily chemical bandage to supposedly keep me going.

Into it I went, in my usual impetuous fashion, and so began my descent into the unknown land of withdrawal from prescription drugs.

The main reason for my writing this book about 'the dark night of my soul' is to document what then took place and my eventual resurrection and to offer you a tangible way out. It's easier to write it now, knowing how everything worked out, but if you can imagine that at that time when I took the plunge, I was living alone, trying to work and still keep some semblance of my life balance going, such as paying the rent, shopping for food and cooking, so when the real madness started, it was pretty tough going.

I realise now when I look back on the massive fallout and effects on my life that I probably came off the Ativan far too quickly and should've had more help, but in the nineties there really was no help on offer so that was not an option.

If I was doing it now, with all the information available on the internet, I would've had a far easier ride if I'd followed the newer protocol of weaning off the Ativan with its short half-life and swinging over onto the long half-life diazepam (Valium) and then slowly coming down off the Valium.

The time frame of the whole process on the Ativan chart to be followed is over 38 weeks, whereas, as you will see as my story unfolds, I stumbled through my total withdrawal over about 16 weeks with no Valium to soften the pain. I've often wondered how the process would've panned out for me if I'd taken longer and swung over to Valium to ease me through. I'll never know.

Sleep deprivation was the first major issue to contend with. I've always been a light sleeper and mild insomnia has been a chronic problem for most of my life. (In fact, it was my search for a good night's sleep that got me into this situation of addiction in the first place.) In what seemed like an eternity but was only the second week of my entering withdrawal, I was already down to being curled up naked in the foetal position on the bedroom floor, as my bed wouldn't stop shaking like a concrete mixer (hallucination) and the hot and cold sweats were crawling all over me like a thousand angry snakes.

Feelings like electric shocks kept running through my arms and legs, along with intense stomach cramps and spasms. My sensitivity to the slightest noise was magnified a thousand times and even a ceiling light would be blinding with glare. A few years back in New Zealand when I'd done a very slow withdrawal over a year, I hadn't experienced anything like the symptoms I got this time around, although I had only got to cutting down to half my dosage in that previous attempt, so I guess that hardly counted as a serious effort.

The next-door neighbour would leave for work around 5am, revving up his motorbike as he went down the nearby driveway, so you can imagine what that was like to my sleep-deprived, jangled senses.

In the next unit in the apartment block in which I was living, there were a bunch of Asian students who would come home around 2 am and proceed to jabber on in what sounded like Chinese whilst they banged and clattered on their woks making up some bloody Asian stir-fry. I told a friend about this, leaving out telling him about the withdrawal process I was going through. In fact, no one knew what I was going through, as shame had always made me keep my addiction a secret.

A slight touch of humour was added to my nightly madness and sleep deprivation when my friend reappeared with a container with what looked like six chicken's feet stuck, talons side up, in some gooey mess, which he left outside the noisy Asians' front door. Apparently, this symbolises terrible bad luck or something similar in Chinese mythology, so when the Asians came jabbering up the internal stairwell at their usual time in the early hours of the morning, there was momentary silence followed by loud yelling and then nothing. Never heard much from them again, so the chicken's feet obviously had the desired effect.

Across the hallway was a weirdo who worked as a TV cameraman and for reasons unknown called himself 'Bat-sucker Bob'. He was a closet gay and a real stoner and would regularly bang on my door, having locked himself out or wanting to borrow money amidst sleazy invitations to come on over to his apartment for some undeclared 'fun'. More frazzled nerves!

So, the daily circus around me really wasn't conducive to a calm and serene place to go through withdrawal, but that was where I was at and it could've been a lot worse. At least, I was basically safe and not far from the General Hospital.

My apartment was only one street back from the main river which snaked through Brisbane City. Many a time I would find myself, after my long day's journey into the night, wandering aimlessly like an urban vampire on the riverbank, feeling nothing but confusion and high anxiety as various harmless joggers and people walking dogs would glide on by, scaring the hell out of me as they appeared like disembodied zombies out of the darkness. One night, whilst out wandering, I ran across an old friend, 'Two Grand' Tony and his lady love. He must've thought there was something very weird going on with me as I tried to reply in a garbled fashion to his questions about how my life was going, before I just freaked out and scuttled off into the night, leaving them standing there. Too much anxiety, too much fear!

14

The self-detox fallout

I really wasn't far into the Ativan withdrawal process and already I was grinding my teeth so badly that further down the line, I had to have a lot of cracked fillings replaced and teeth crowned.

The serious vomiting and retching had started kicking in around week three, even though I wasn't eating much. I can remember being in a cold shower in the middle of the night, bathed in sweat, trying to cool down and projectile vomiting all over the shower walls at the same time. But I kept going.

My brain felt like it was melting and running out my ears, whilst those continuous spasms and twitches appeared all over my face and legs and I'd only just begun to withdraw. You couldn't make this stuff up. How bad was it going to get?

I came to dread the nightly horror movie as I tried to get some sleep. When I did drift into a half sleep in the twilight zone, I had terrible nightmares about being crushed by giant objects like a huge ship plunging me under the waves and can recall one time waking up, jabbering parts of the Lord's Prayer as if to try to banish the demons swirling around me like angry wraiths. It did occur to me that my very survival was being threatened, as I sailed into these uncharted waters of my core being, and that I may not come out the other side, due to my body shutting down completely. This may sound dramatic, but it does happen.

But I kept going.

Reading this you may be thinking, why did he keep going?

I guess, as I said earlier, I have a very strong will and something deep inside me that guides me on. So, I carried on stumbling my way onwards whilst slowly shaving down the dreaded pills. I knew instinctively that if I didn't get clean this time from this addiction, my life was that of a chemical slave and that ain't me, babe!

As far as I was concerned, my brain chemistry and nervous system had been damaged by the benzo chemicals I had taken for the previous 13 years and the challenge ahead was to try to repair myself. That wasn't going to be easy or achieved overnight, so I was well aware of the unpleasant fact that I was in it for the long haul.

Meanwhile, during the day, I tried to keep working and do my sales calls to large corporate clients. All I had to keep me aimed in the right direction was a well-honed, inner marketing, verbal template that had served me well in the past allowing me to make my way through the face-to-face appointments. Amazingly, I was still managing to generate business but the anxiety levels by now were phenomenal as the supply of GABA from the benzos started to dry up in my brain. Everything then becomes magnified to an extreme level of fear or paranoia, when it's just a harmless everyday event for most people.

If you've ever seen that famous painting by Edvard Munch, *The Scream*, then you'll know what I'm talking about. Imagine being in the heart of the city, surrounded by cars speeding past, jangling noises everywhere, traffic lights flashing, surging crowds of people pressing in all around you and an overwhelming agoraphobic fear of life crushing your very being, then you may have a slight idea of what it was like for me to try to maintain a work and appointment schedule. Near on impossible. But I kept going.

I was speeding through two or three business shirts a day as the anxiety sweats and the Queensland heat soaked me through to my skin. I'd carry a change of kit in the car and after an appointment I would duck into a car park toilet and do my Clark Kent–Superman change of uniform and then off to another appointment. As Winston Churchill famously said, 'If you're going through hell, keep going!'

Some very strange hallucinations would momentarily appear, mostly of the negative kind, but I do clearly remember a very surreal experience one hot summer's afternoon. I'd gone home to try to get some rest. I was lying naked on my bed in a sort of half daze from the humidity, coincidentally listening to Patsy Cline singing 'Crazy' on the player, when I genuinely felt this great calm come over me and the sense of something like a large, white being of an angelic vibe landing ever so softly on my body and spreading its metaphorical wings all over me, engendering a precious moment of cool peace and then it was gone!

I think you must believe that sometimes you're on the side of the angels when you're trying to do the right thing. I don't know what this ethereal apparition was but I was deeply grateful for that fleeting moment of spiritual respite.

I had a good friend at that time who, luckily for me, had been through a milder version of what I was going through, so she was able to keep me bolstered and offer me solace at her house when the madness got too much, but it was of little comfort, as it was my whole being that was flying to pieces, not hers.

In my daily life, even the smallest of tasks took on gigantic proportions. I kept doing forgetful things such as leaving tap's running and overflowing the kitchen sink as I wandered around my apartment mumbling to myself, along with events like nearly electrocuting myself plugging in the coffee jug. When the phone rang, I would just stare at it in terror until it stopped ringing and you could forget about knocking on the apartment door. I was never at home in my head.

In a slightly humorous but unfortunate vein, one hot and sticky night I ended up being arrested by the vicious Queensland cops, who have no hesitation in giving you a beating and throwing you in jail for the night. What happened was that I'd gone somewhere and ended up coming home drunk. Because of the heat, I'd stripped down to my underpants, poured a drink and turned up the volume on my stereo whilst strolling around my abode, wearing my straw cowboy hat.

A bunch of pretty nurses on the level below in the apartment block complained to the cops and next thing I'm being confronted by two young patrolmen wandering around my apartment and giving me the third degree. I started jabbering on about my rights and in a flash, I'm handcuffed. Ranting about coming off medication seemed to only amuse them, as did my odd attire of near nakedness and a cowboy hat.

After letting me get dressed, they took me downtown in a patrol car and threw me in a cell, only letting me go as the sun was coming up. I got home and crashed into an alcoholic sleep, but somewhere in my tired, inebriated brain, I forgot that they had given me a summons to turn up at the Magistrates Court later that morning, for being a public nuisance.

By the time I awoke, it was nearly midday. I saw the summons on the kitchen bench, so I grabbed a cab and hotfooted it to the court. The judge had just seen his last case and was leaving for the day, so he wasn't impressed at having to be called back. He made this clear by fining me A$250. Unfortunately, this episode activated my current address in the police database, so for the next few weeks a flurry of old unpaid parking tickets kept arriving in the mail, which I could ill-afford to pay and only added another level of misery to my daily existence.

15

Now for the crazy stuff

Another thing that I hadn't considered when I started self-detoxing was that my hand-eye co-ordination and all my spatial reactions in my brain had been altered and recalibrated over the years by the numbing of the GABA receptors in my cerebral cortex due to the benzos, so as I emerged out of dependency, things were incrementally and very slightly different each day and driving was one of the most noticeable. Every new day, I had to adjust to a slight change in perception.

The straw that broke the camel's back was when I crashed my car, which I'd already managed to sideswipe backing out of the apartment garage due to the spatial distortion.

On this Saturday afternoon, I was driving to see a friend when I entered a line of cars waiting for the traffic lights to change. We got a green and they all moved forward and then some fool further up the line chose to stop, causing everyone to brake, but because my reactions were out of kilter, I ploughed straight into the back of the car in front of me.

Given my anxiety levels, I just fell to pieces, shaking like a leaf, but fortunately the driver I had rammed into assumed I was simply in shock and took my details, got the car towed to the panel shop and somehow, I got home.

I could go on and on about all the debilitating symptoms and hassles that occurred over those early months of self-detox and there were many, many more, but to describe them all would only serve to frighten you and the idea is to encourage you take the same steps as me and free yourself from chemical dependency. I see absolutely no point in writing a 'misery memoir' full of terrifying doom and gloom without offering you any bright, future prospects. What's the point in my documenting pages and pages of terrible things that happened to me which would only serve to put you off ever considering taking the steps to be free of your own personal chemical addiction? Suffice to say it was a very harrowing time and experience.

Sleep deprivation at the best of times can make you psychotic, but in my case, I went, at one stage, nearly six days without sleep. I found myself sitting in a public park one sunny afternoon, gripped in fear and experiencing what felt like some sort of separate reality, which I guess was a psychosis of sorts.

People were walking around me, going about their everyday business of playing fetch with their dog, picnicking with their children and generally having a cruisy day, but to me it was like being in a parallel universe under the influence of a psychedelic.

Maybe I was psychotic in that moment and I can see how

I could've easily lost it, as I was so close to the edge at that time. It's quite possible that I could've flipped out and ended up in bad trouble with the dreaded authorities, so I thank my inner resources that kept me going that day and helped me find my way back to my apartment in my freshly repaired car.

When I talk about those days of withdrawal madness, I'm glad that I'd had the past experiences that go with smoking very strong ganja (marijuana). Back in the seventies in New Zealand there was a lot of what they called 'Buddha sticks' floating around, imported from Thailand, courtesy of the notorious Mr Asia gang.

This weed was exceptionally potent, like skunk sinsemilla, and you could have some rather unpleasant paranoid times on it, but what you did learn very quickly was that the scary times always went away and the good times reappeared when the stoned inner-world levelled out. So, no matter how weird things got during those early withdrawal days in Brisbane, I had that ability, based on prior knowledge, to separate myself into the experiencer watching the experience. Nowadays they call it 'mindfulness'.

I have since read latterly available material on withdrawal and as I said earlier, in hindsight, I think that I cut down on my Ativan far too quickly. The conventional wisdom nowadays is that the procedure that I should've followed was to swing over from the Ativan and go onto a starting point of an equivalent 30–50 milligrams of Valium a day for a while and then taper down off the Valium over time.

Ativan's very short half-life in your system means it doesn't take long before you enter a withdrawal state. Valium stays in your body for considerably longer with a reported half-life per pill of up to 200 hours, which gives your receptors plenty of time to adjust to your withdrawal regime. I was, unfortunately, unaware of this crucial factor and had no one to advise me. I was just keen to rid my system of Ativan but I probably could've saved myself a lot of mental torture and grief if I had known about it.

I can't be sure of the months or the dates during that withdrawal time but I think, when I finally got down to taking nothing, zilch, no pills, it was about the third or fourth month after starting from day one, so it was probably sometime around the end of April. Throughout this process, I'd loosely kept in touch with the shrink, Dr Zed, whom I talked about earlier. He still hadn't ever discussed with me the prospect of stopping taking benzos and had always given me prescriptions, so when I was spinning out in the early withdrawal stages, he'd usually given me some loose advice over the phone when I'd ring him jabbering on about going crazy. However, once again my blind faith in the medical profession was about to deliver me another breach of trust, courtesy of good old Dr Zed.

It's too hard for me to convey here in writing quite how my mental state was after around four months of hell, as I was running on empty from a cocktail of withdrawal, lack of sleep, serious loss of weight, etc., but I had rung in a panic and made an appointment with Dr Zed.

When I got down to his consulting rooms on the Gold Coast, I told him how I felt and the terrible withdrawal symptoms I'd been going through for weeks and weeks. He soothingly convinced me that my brain was malfunctioning from lack of its daily chemical benzo pill and that was fine and that giving up tranquillisers was admirable and what a hero I was for coming this far. But it didn't have to be this hard, Rob! Why suffer needlessly?

Yessirree, he had just come from a medical conference (probably in Transylvania) and, wonder of wonders, he had some samples of this new miracle drug that I can distinctly recall him describing as 'the champagne of all modern drugs' and that I should give them a try.

He promised me that they were definitely not dependency forming and that, after only a short period of usage, they would effortlessly walk me back to a calm and fruitful life. Imagine that. Free at last!

16

My 'shrink' betrays me

'Doctors have throughout time made fortunes on killing their patients with their cures. The difference in psychiatry is that it is the death of the soul.'
— RD Laing

In my frazzled state of mind, like a suicide bomber believing that martyrdom would take him to paradise with 70 virgins, I fell for it all over again just as I had back in New Zealand with that crazy bastard Dr Dan.

Dr Zed, the man whose home I had visited for meals, whom I had bared my inner soul to over the last couple of years and whom I had trusted, was now giving me a drug that turned out to be highly addictive and responsible for many users committing suicide, at the worst.

Aropax (or paroxetine) was its name and it came in a nice, shiny silver strip with bluebirds on the packet. Of course it did!

What he was giving me was one of the first new waves of SSRI (selective serotonin reuptake inhibitor) antidepressant pills (Prozac was of the same breed and came soon after, as fluoxetine).

I may have been understandably feeling down mentally due to the prior months of withdrawal chaos and was probably exhibiting signs of reactive depression to everything, but the nature of the drugs he was peddling was once again not explained to me and definitely not appropriate to my circumstances. I was simply told everything was going to be cool and that I'd be sleeping like a baby again, courtesy of the good doctor.

Back then I didn't have the technology available, as I do now, to check what Aropax was but the following details are easily found online nowadays. There are many documented side effects to the drug, including these:

Like other antidepressants, paroxetine (Aropax) may increase the risk of suicidal thinking and behaviour in children and adolescents. The FDA conducted a statistical analysis of paroxetine (Aropax) clinical trials in children and adolescents, finding an increase in 'suicidality' and ideation as compared to placebo; the trend for increased 'suicidality' was observed in both trials for depression and for anxiety disorders.

Many psychoactive medications can cause withdrawal symptoms among the highest incidence rates and severity of withdrawal syndrome of any medication of its class. Common withdrawal symptoms for paroxetine include nausea, dizziness, light-headedness and vertigo; insomnia, nightmares and vivid dreams; feelings of electricity in the body, as well as crying and anxiety upon discontinuation from administration. Evidence has shown that paroxetine also has among the highest incidence rates and severity of withdrawal syndrome of any medication of its class.

I can't really explain why I fell for it. I guess I was just so tired of fighting the pain of weeks of withdrawal that I simply wanted a break from the madness going on around and inside me. Plus, I trusted him. I don't really know the answer but that night I took the Aropax, courtesy of Dr Zed.

Some things on the road of life make a sudden 180-degree turn in altering your direction, and this was one of those moments.

Within two days, I was off the planet but in a very dangerous and bad way. My poor old brain had only just fought its way to a sort of chemical semi-freedom in withdrawing from Ativan and now, marching down the neural highway was a fresh, new pharmaceutical army looking to find a home in my cranial receptors. And they sure did, plugging into any random socket or receptor available. What a hell night that was! Bigger than December'63 or the night they drove old Dixie down, for sure.

Totally off the wall, I rang my friends Frank and Ava down over the border, raving like a chimpanzee. I guess they wondered what was going on as I'd never told them anything about benzos, Dr Zed, withdrawal, etc. All they knew was that I was a good mate who liked to party, so they immediately insisted that I come down and stay with them and let them know what the hell was happening?

Within hours, the sinister potential side effect of Aropax was already manifesting itself in the form of a strongly unreasonable compulsion to kill myself! As outlined above, this can be a well-documented side effect of SSRI's and many a person has inexplicably topped himself or herself as soon as they've started taking them.

Sixties American pop star Del Shannon was a famous case in point. His career was on the comeback trail and he was doing fine but was prescribed Prozac and after just two weeks of taking the drug, he blew his brains out in his Santa Clarita home in California on Feb 3, 1990 causing his widow to file a lawsuit against the drug company who were the makers of Prozac. There are many more documented examples of similar suicides. The recent death of a Chicago attorney who committed suicide by jumping under a train was allegedly caused by the generic version of an antidepressant medication that he was taking, according to a federal jury in Chicago, which ordered drug giant GlaxoSmithKline (GSK) to pay $3 million to his widow.

The jury found GSK liable for the death of Stewart Dolin, who jumped in front of a Blue Line train in the Loop in July 2010. In April 2017, the jury awarded Wendy Dolin $2 million in damages and $1 million for her husband's suffering, according to the law firm representing her in US District Court in Chicago.

Because of this growing, seductive death imagery in my mind, I was starting to really spin like the proverbial top and panic attacks were swarming in. Not only was I in detox withdrawal from one drug, but now my psyche was also trying to contend with new chemicals and a whole raft of other life-threatening ideations.

In the morning, I rang Dr Zed in a state of very high anxiety and made an appointment to see him on the way down the coast to my friends Frank and Ava. At the same time, for some strange reason, I had made an appointment to get my hair cut by the hairdresser I regularly visited down in Surfers Paradise, where Dr Zed also held court.

After the haircut, the hairdresser held the mirror up so I could check how much hair he'd clipped off the back. When I looked in the mirror all I saw was a distorted hallucination of the back of my head being blown away by, I guess, a shotgun in a suicide attempt. Sounds weird but it's true.

The Gold Coast sun was beating down under azure blue skies and holidaymakers were happily scurrying everywhere around me, but I was so depersonalised and frightened by now that I hardly knew where I was.

I fled from the hairdressing salon in terror and straight up to the nearby surgery of Dr Zed and as soon as I got into his consulting room, I disintegrated.

Fell into a million pieces!

Bits of what was left of me shattered like flying shards of psychic breaking glass, all over his consulting room floor, landing here and there and then back over here. All the months of withdrawal and years of lack of inner child resolution, in fact my whole life, finally caught up with me and my reserves just folded up. I threw in the towel, collapsing on his clinic floor and curling up in a sobbing, heaving mess whilst he sat silently watching. I can remember muttering 'Am I having a nervous breakdown?', to which he casually replied 'Probably.'

I don't recall much conversation between us after that but he seemed to indicate that maybe Aropax wasn't quite the champagne drug for this poor boy after all, and that what he now recommended was a short stay in a nearby, very expensive private hospital, akin to the Betty Ford clinic in the States.

It was now late afternoon and to check in this late in the day, he said, was a waste of good money as the day was half over, so he decided that he would very considerately let me sleep on the couch in his clinic's waiting room for the night, which would save me money and then we could get this hospital thing sorted out the next day.

I marvel now at such weird logic because I could've gone berserk and wrecked his clinic during the night, but I went along with it because by that time, I was too far gone to care and had pretty much reverted to a sort of catatonia. I spent that night alone in a shrink's clinic on the Gold Coast of Australia, spinning like a top and half out of my mind with no direction home!

What had happened to me, I wondered, and to all my good intentions that had, once again, been hijacked by the pharmaceutical industry? Needless to say, I saw the dawn coming up without having had much sleep.

17

———

Cuckoo's nest and golden beaches

The new day saw things get even crazier. Because the hospital was so expensive they needed to have the bill guaranteed, so Dr Zed rang my older brother in New Zealand, who knew nothing about my benzo dependency and 'shrinks'.

You can imagine my brother's surprise to hear a hitherto unknown shrink on the Gold Coast of Australia explaining the reason for the call being the need for a financial guarantee of payment for a hospital bill, before passing me the phone. I took up the phone but immediately started sobbing and mumbling gibberish nonsense, which set my brother off. Between our mutual sobbing, he guaranteed the bill and said he'd be on the next flight over from New Zealand.

As an aside, I read years later of a young woman who found herself having intrusive thoughts of killing herself, such as I had, so she'd written a suicide note and brought it with her to her psychiatrist.

Standard procedure for a therapist when a client brings up suicide is to admit them to a hospital (in large part to avoid being held responsible for negligence, should the person commit suicide). So, the psychiatrist drove the poor woman to a hospital to check her in.

But along the way, he had her stop at an ATM machine to extract the money to pay for her last visit — so that if she had gone through with her suicidal ideation and killed herself, the psychiatrist would not have been out of pocket for the expense of her final session. It was not until months later that the woman regained enough cognitive ability to realise that the doctor's treatment of her had been somewhat monstrous.

Sounds familiar but you've got to see the gallows humour in it, I guess.

My arrival at the high-class hospital was like something out of *One Flew Over the Cuckoo's Nest*. Doctor Zed spoke to the white-coated people in the plush foyer, who all nodded knowingly, whilst I sat huddled like Randle.P. McMurphy (Jack Nicholson) in the waiting room. Next thing I knew I was in a luxurious private suite, laid out on a bed and slammed full of God knows what, which they injected into me, and then they apparently put me on a politely subtle suicide watch.

Because I was originally heading south to see my friends, I conveniently had my toiletries packed in my overnight bag in my car, but they took that off me and reassuringly removed my shaving gear and anything else remotely likely to be used to 'off' myself. Death by toothbrush. Very dangerous.

I lay in a torpor for most of that day and the craziness

continued when hospital staff turned up in the evening to present me with the dinner menu, which had options like braised Californian quail with baby roast potatoes and sautéed scarlet beans or freshly smoked salmon encased in a light filo pastry. Too much for this kid. I chose the quail and not long afterwards a white-coated nurse came and gave me some type of pill to knock me out. Next thing I knew it was a brand-new day and I was awakening to find my New Zealand, older brother standing by my bed.

I stayed, I think, for three nights there and then checked out, minus about an A$1800 bill for my stay, and my brother and I limped back to my apartment in Brisbane in my car.

I never saw Dr Zed again and had no desire to. Even in my numbed state, I realised that I had been callously used to test out a new pharmaceutical company drug and I'm sure my adverse reaction was written up in some medical report filed with 'subject A' did not respond well!

Dr Zed had filled a prescription for me for one of the drugs they'd plugged into me in the hospital, which was an older drug called Doxepin (apparently an antidepressant), with the instructions to take three pills daily, which was the standard dose of 150 milligrams.

Given that recent research globally has come up with the factoid that up to 40% of antidepressant users get no benefit from the drug they're prescribed when compared with placebo users in clinical trials, it's hard to know what the pills he prescribed were meant to be doing to me, but taking them only added to my feeling of mental and physical numbness, combined with a stronger than usual sense of hopelessness.

Here I was again, having gone through more horror over

the last week and months and all it had led me to was ending up on another drug called Doxepin which, a few months further down the track, I sensibly dumped without much drama or fallout but the good news was (always look for the silver lining) that throughout everything, I was no longer taking benzos, which was my original mission, and this was a very big deal to me, having come this far. Progress was being made even if it was only baby steps.

When we arrived back in Brisbane, my older brother, who has a tendency towards a love of bureaucracy, swung into gear and within 24 hours had me traipsing around behind him like a puppy, dazed and confused and in a state of numbness, as we visited various government drug and alcohol agencies in the city. I think his intention was to get me looped into the system so that he could fly back to New Zealand knowing some starting point for me had been sorted out, which was sensible, I suppose.

After filing my name and details with some faceless bureaucrat at the Biala Drug and Alcohol Centre in Roma Street in the CBD, we went up in the afternoon to a lookout on Mt Coot-tha, overlooking Brisbane City, and I can clearly remember turning to my him and saying, 'I don't know how I'm ever going to come back from this or even survive.' A terrible bleakness seeped into every part of my mind, and death seemed an increasingly viable option.

Try to imagine what it was like after months of withdrawal and holding on to my sanity and now being confronted with being alone, no future prospects and all normal mental defences down and in disarray. Not good!

A couple of days later, my brother flew back to New Zealand, but not before he'd got our mutual friend, Frank from South Golden Beach, to come up from over the New South Wales state border and take the reins. Fortunately, we all knew each other from our teenage days flatting together in New Zealand, and Frank gave my brother the firm assurance that he'd look after me until I was able to look after myself.

I said goodbye to my brother, locked up my apartment and with Frank driving slowly behind me along the freeway, we took about four hours to do what should have been a two-hour trip from Brisbane to south of the Queensland border. My extreme anxiety levels in the busy southern motorway traffic as cars sped past me like manic wasps, were of such an amplified magnitude that I could only crawl along at a snail's pace in the slow lane with angry motorists honking at me and shaking their fists as they overtook me, till we finally made it to South Golden Beach.

My friends installed me in the loft above the garage, which was separate from their main house, and this was to be my bolt hole for the next six months or so. I'd stayed in the loft many times back in the party days, but the party lights had been turned off and now I was just a badly broken human being in an altered state of mind.

Scrambled brains, jobless and damn near out of money, and the only things to show for my life being a car, a clothes rack and two large cardboard cartons containing my worldly goods.

Everything else either was still locked up in my apartment in Brisbane, which didn't amount to a lot, or had vanished into the slipstream of my life during my abortive trip to the UK. Given I'd migrated there, supposedly for good, I'd sold a lot of my stuff before going.

Frank and Ava were extremely kind to me, but naturally their everyday boozey lifestyle still carried on. So here we have a mega-anxious me skulking around the place with my constantly dry mouth hanging open like some looney that had escaped from Nurse Ratched at Cuckoos-ville, a large standard poodle called Hugo for company and my friends bouncing off the walls each weekend on rum or bubbly wine. Like most of those days during withdrawal, the word 'surreal' hardly covered describing what was going on in my daily view of the world.

Within days, the government system, previously activated in Brisbane by my brother, rolled into place with a phone call from a calm-sounding woman called Jane, who informed me that she was a drug and alcohol counsellor from a nearby local hospital at Mullumbimby. She set up an appointment to come over to the beach house to see me the next day and when she duly arrived, turned out to be a very laid-back, pleasant-looking woman who shook my hand with a warm greeting and the magic words: 'Don't worry. I've been where you are and we'll get things sorted out for you.' And then, 'It does get better, I can guarantee you that.'

Unbelievable! You can't begin to imagine what it felt like to hear those words. Talk about a life raft. Hope had arrived! She explained that she had also been through the withdrawal experience that I was suffering, before becoming a counsellor, so I was in safe hands.

At last! I'd finally found someone who understood what I was having to endure and apparently had the tools at her disposal to point me in the right direction. And, although she was from the Drug and Alcohol annex of the local hospital, she was not a bloody doctor whose only ambition was to fit me up with more drugs to further blow my mind.

18

Hallucinations, poodles and dolphins

I made a time to go and see her the following week and then lapsed back into my usual state of the spin cycle in my mind being set on 'high'. Part of the arrangement I had with my friends where I was staying was that I would look after the beach house and walk their poodle, Hugo, each day whilst they commuted back up over the border to Brisbane for their work week. Frank had his own import business and Ava was high up the feed chain in some advertising agency.

Given my fragile state of mind, I was probably somewhat unsafe to be left alone in their beach house on the east coast of Australia, like Quoyle out of Annie Proulx's award-winning book *The Shipping News* (if you've read the book or seen the movie, you'll know what I mean), but I wasn't about to argue, being grateful for all small mercies that came my way.

Each morning, under the hot sun, I'd walk Hugo at a slow pace up the long, golden beach, burning up my limited energy levels. It wasn't too bad really, as often surfing along beside us would be pods of dolphins framed in the waves, happily living in the moment, whilst out in the bay, humpback whales would breach high out of the water as they headed north to their traditional mating grounds.

However, things such as Hugo slipping his leash and disappearing into the sandhills with me staggering after him could very easily trigger mega-panic within me. In an instant, my brain would flood my system with cortisol and adrenaline as I flashed through an imaginary sequence of events, entailing me losing the dog and being lashed to the yardarm, whipped and banished by Frank and Ava when they got home. Given Ava's temperament, that was always a distinct possibility, but these heightened threats to what little security I had left in my life were a constant, daily drama one way or another.

Because my anxiety was ratcheted so high from the starvation of natural chemicals in my brain, something like losing the dog would take on gigantic proportions way beyond what the situation required, and would trigger an anxiety attack.

Putting concepts together rapidly, such as thinking how to catch a vanished dog, was hampered by my brain's synapses and neural pathways getting tangled up on go-slow, so when I'd eventually catch up with Hugo and put him back on the lead, I'd just sit on a sand hill staring out to sea, with the tears rolling down my cheeks like a grateful virgin.

It pays to remember that although it seems like an eternity at the actual time, in reality, an anxiety episode usually only lasts 20 to 30 seconds, so if you can remember that, then you won't get anxious about being anxious when you next get anxious? (Smile now)

Insomnia was still a major issue for me and most nights up in the loft would find me in the early hours of the morning cupping my hands over my face and recycling my breathing or blowing into a paper bag, which had the known side effect of lowering the hyperventilation that had pumped too much oxygen into my bloodstream, inducing an anxiety hit.

A couple of times my heart was racing so fast and palpitating like I had boulders bouncing around in my chest, I was convinced I was having a heart attack or a stroke and thought I was going to have to call an ambulance, which would've been a waste of time as the nearest ambulance station was an hour away down the coast at Byron Bay. I would've been dead by the time they got to me. Bear in mind, five days out of seven, I was alone at the beach house so there was no one to call for help.

Terrible dreams and nightmares are a well-known side effect of benzo withdrawal and in the TRANX brochures they refer to some normal, heterosexual, married men, whilst going through withdrawal, committing suicide after experiencing, repetitively, vivid dreams of having sex with other men or with their daughters, which was completely contrary to their nature.

Can't say any of that happened to me but I had some very disturbing dreams oozing up from the primal swamp of my subconscious mind containing a surreal, chaotic mixture of real and imaginary instances of my earlier life, which would wake me up in a cold sweat. Night sweats were a very regular feature, so a towel was always on standby.

I remember with great clarity a very weird hallucination I had one dark night alone up there in the loft.

I was immersed in a nightmare which appeared to be about me being somewhere in a dark mountain valley that looked like something out of *Game of Thrones*. All around me were wispy demons and witch-like crones and creatures. There seemed to be some rant going on about the chemical symbols for minerals whilst I was being sucked down a vortex-like, long, rocky crevice. The witch women were all trying to pull at my limbs and I was sinking into darkness and oblivion. I struggled out of this and woke up with a start and looked by my bedside table.

There, shimmering in the dark beside me, was something that looked like the portal you'd see on the *Stargate* movies and in the centre, shifting in shape like a hologram, was Anubis, a distorted, dog-like creature of some kind. Realising it was a hallucination, I was morbidly fascinated for the few seconds that it sat beside me, like a menacing luminous blob, and then it vanished.

Maybe it was my subconscious version of Hugo the poodle wanting to take a walk on the wild side in the middle of the night, but I somehow doubt that. I had a couple of other hallucinations further on which I'll get to but, fortunately (or maybe unfortunately?), hallucinations were not a large part of my withdrawal and recovery process.

I think now is a good time to point out that not everybody who takes benzodiazepines suffers what I and many others have gone through in the withdrawal process. Usually those lucky ones who get a free ride are the ones who don't stay on them for a long time, but it's a proven fact that taking benzo tranquillisers for as short a time as three weeks can lock you into an addiction.

To give you a documented example of current prescribing rates in my small country of New Zealand, here are some official statistics up to 2013 from Pharmac, which is the New Zealand drug-buying agency.

2004: anxiolytics (benzodiazepine group), 293,500 prescriptions

2013: 371,700, which is an increase of 26%

2004: sedatives and hypnotics (sleepers like Zoplicone), 521,300

2013: 703,700, which is an increase of 35%

2004: SSRI antidepressants, 541,400

2013: 860,200, which is an increase of 59%

Bearing in mind that New Zealand has only a small population base of under five million, that's a huge amount of increased prescribing by doctors over the last decade of drugs that are potentially addictive, with well-documented side effects and have ruined many lives. You can multiply these figures up into the many millions, annually, when you look at the same statistics for places like the US and the UK. So why are governments around the world, including mine, allowing this to go on?

In January of 2004, a communication from the Chief Medical Officer in the UK to all doctors nationally reaffirmed the addiction position with a 'Benzodiazepines Warning' concerning patient safety:

Doctors are being reminded that benzodiazepines should only be prescribed for short-term treatment, in light of continued reports about problems with long-term use.

The European Union's guidelines to the medical profession (volume 3b) stated it even more definitively:

> *Use of benzodiazepines may lead to the development of physical and psychic dependence upon these products. The risk of dependence increases with dose and duration of treatment.*
>
> *The duration of treatment should be as short as possible, depending on the indication, but should not exceed four weeks for insomnia and eight to twelve weeks for anxiety, including the tapering off process.*
>
> *Extension beyond these periods should not take place without re-evaluation of the situation.*
>
> *In fact, not only does use of benzodiazepines beyond these time periods increase the risk of dependence, there is evidence that the very effectiveness of the drugs to treat patients' problems for more than a short time is dubious.*

But still doctors keep prescribing them, repeatedly, to the same patients. Some doctors I've spoken to defend the issuing of benzo scripts as being helpful in certain circumstances such as grief or high stress, and I'm sure this is true, but when a doctor continues to prescribe beyond the notified safety limit of around four weeks to the same person, then that is negligence, in my opinion, and the beginning of the creation of an addict.

19

Madness, counsellors and suicide

I'd started my detox and tapering withdrawal in January and it was now the month of May, so I'd been completely free of the benzos in my system for only a few weeks from the initial day one of entering withdrawal.

One thing they did tell me at TRANX was that the rule of thumb is that it takes six months for every year you've been addicted, to get the drug residue out of your system.

Knowing there was the possibility that I'd keep experiencing various withdrawal symptoms ongoing for that many years to come seemed just another cruel burden. But personally, that suggested formula didn't turn out that way for me.

But if you've ever given up smoking (and I had), you'll be able to relate to how long it takes to be free of the cravings for a cigarette, so, one way another, you must pay the piper for your past choices or misfortunes.

Its a strange irony that we all long for a lazy holiday by the beach away from our daily stresses, yet here I was, stranded in paradise, stressed to the max, with no sign of anything vaguely resembling a holiday. Under a different set of circumstances, it would have been amazing. The beautiful blue skies each day and the blazing sun beating down with the sounds of the rolling ocean nearby would be most people's dream life. However, I wasn't living that dream life but actually going slowly mad with withdrawal and anxious uncertainty.

Fortunately, Jane, my new-found friend and drug and alcohol counsellor, had things under control and within a week or so, I found myself sitting across her desk at my first official appointment in the drug and alcohol section of the Mullumbimby Hospital, which was not too far away from where I was currently living. I should point out that this was not your high-end hospital, just a small-town, country version, but it appeared to be clean and efficient.

Because Byron Bay and its nearby environs, like Nimbin and Mullumbimby, are the Mecca for the hippie and drug culture from all over Australia, there were plenty of support services available (and, of course, street drugs of every persuasion).

I honestly can't remember what Jane had to offer other than understanding conversation, friendship and a handful of brochures, but that was enough to give me some point of reference to hang on to, plus her mental nourishment by being a friendly face.

When I first arrived down from Brisbane to Frank and Ava's house by the beach, my world had become sealed over with a grey, bleak film of high anxiety, depression and hopelessness, but as my Gods pointed me to people like Jane, a small window appeared in the attic of my mind and I knew that if I held on long enough and followed my instincts, I could slowly reverse my way out of this desperate hole that I'd fallen into and that the tiny window of my inner world would slowly expand to become a brighter picture.

You've no doubt heard of Pandora's box? Well, this was sort of like Pandora's box in reverse and I guess you know what they found at the bottom of Pandora's box after all the demons had fled? Hope, and hope was about all I had left to hang on to.

They say that the ancient Greek tales of mythology, like Homer's 'Odyssey', are really hidden blueprints for psychological travails of the mind and soul, cleverly disguising what happens during a mental breakdown. When you think about Homer's descriptions of the sailors being lured onto the rocks by the Sirens, etc., and then Odysseus/Ulysses eventually finding his way 'home' to Penelope/Persephone (sanity) whilst under the protection of the goddess Athena, it's not hard to correlate that ancient mythology with what I was going through.

When you're under the pump with most systems flashing red, you hang on to any intelligent concept you can find; be it mythology, books or bullshit, as you bob along feeling like you're completely alone, miles out to sea, swimming for dear life but not knowing where the shore is.

Because I believe in karma, synchronicity and the laws of serendipity, I had enough occult and esoteric knowledge to be able to 'read the tea leaves' and baby-step my way through some of the madness swirling around me, but I'm not sure how a person would get on who really had no strong belief system. Everything you've ever wanted is on the other side of fear, but the trick is to figure out how to get rid of the current fear that riddles your every pore, so you can get to that mirage-like other side. Not easy.

My Ativan-free days trickled by as I entered deeply into what I was totally unprepared for and that was the emotional withdrawal, stage two. When I made the decision to eliminate the Ativan from my life, I assumed that I'd be in for the rough ride of the initial withdrawal (which I certainly got). I was prepared to tough out the highs and lows and then, naïvely, I thought that would be it. A few hard months and the Ativan would be gone and I could get on with my life, minus my daily curse. But nothing prepared me for what happened when the pills were no longer in my nervous system, providing me with a daily chemical bandage over my subconscious psyche and emotions bank.

It is not enough to give up the booze or drugs. That is only the start. It's when the hard work of learning to live back in everyday reality begins, minus the crutch of drugs or alcohol, that life can become such a nightmare. Many get through the initial physical detox period only to run screaming back to the pills or booze when the new emotional reality comes knocking, offering nothing but the naked truth about yourself!

Emotional withdrawal, stage two, is where you get to meet your nasty little ego, which is also fighting for its own survival and is a distorted version of your real self, and it can go on for months or even years.

In my case, all the emotional and unresolved issues I'd had over the previous 13 years of my pill intake and prior (and there were many) had been stuffed deep into the 'rubbish tin' of my mind during that period. Now, with the pills gone and the chemical bandage thrown in the trash can, the lid came flying off my personal Pandora's box and the demons, past hurts, imaginary fears and mislabelled emotions came powering up like a great white shark from the depths of my subconscious ocean and into my consciousness at a time when I was pretty much defenceless and incapable of processing them. Thirteen years and a lifetime is a lot to process, I can assure you, and now The Dark Shadow at the bottom of my rubbish bin was angry. Very angry!

Along with this madness, the seductive whispering of suicide literally became my daily companion to the point that it turned into a game between me, myself and I. Every day, whilst out aimlessly driving around the coast trying to fill in the hours, I'd drive up bush tracks or into remote parks and think to myself, 'Hmm, this looks like a good place to kill myself', and I'd do the mental exercise of which particular method I'd use and what to write as a farewell note.

The old standard of carbon monoxide from the car exhaust usually won, or otherwise poisoning myself with some exotic but deadly tropical flowers taking second billing. The game would then move on to 'Well, if I can find this place or serene spot today, maybe I'll see if I can find an even better spot tomorrow!' And so, it would go on every day for months and months.

This sounds totally pathetic when I recall it, but suicidal ideation seemed to be one of the major side effects of withdrawal stage two. The process that leads people to take their own life and the whispering seduction from your mind to go ahead and do it is driven by the ego down there in the control room. Detecting that its perceived world, which it has taken so many years to create, is now being tortured and threatened with destruction, causes the ego to go into over-drive to protect itself at all cost and to the ego, suicide is a misguided form of self-protection!

Hence the constant whispering rationalising to take your-self out, to self-murder your being, rides with you like a gremlin every waking minute. What the threatened ego doesn't realise, because it's not at a conscious level, is that if the human being kills itself, the ego dies with it.

That's why it'd be more accurate for it to be called 'ego-cide' rather than self-murder or suicide. It is a terrible thing to do to your poor old human 'being' which has carried you through your life, to just selfishly terminate yourself, but that attitude belongs to the land of rational thinking, which is not where the person battling suicidal impulses is in their mind.

So many people judge the suicide victim and waffle on about how selfish they are but that judgment is made by peo-ple who are not in the same state of mind as the suicide vic-tim. How can you judge their hell that made them do it, from your own pleasant little point of view? If anyone is being selfish, it's those who judge! Sometimes I wonder if it's not just the soul writing its own mythology around the path that has led you to the point of stepping into death as the soul considers breaking out for higher ground and departing this mortal coil?

There are far better ways than death, such as mindfulness and meditation, to bring the ego under control, but when you're in the mental state that I was in, this way of thinking seemed very remote. Fortunately, my own higher self was stronger than the suicidal ideation. There were only a few times when I really thought I would go through with it. As they say, suicide is a permanent solution to a temporary problem!

I think it's very important at this point to make a clarification regarding my constant compulsion to commit suicide, because I don't see my situation as that of the normal criteria around suicide. Usually, people that commit suicide leave notes indicating that they've come to the incorrect conclusion that their loved ones would be better off without them being around and that they feel they are just a drag on everyone and better gone from this world. Others have mental disorders, such as paranoid schizophrenia, where they perceive that they're hearing voices from the radio or the devil guiding them to do terrible things, including killing themselves or those around them.

This wasn't the case with my constant suicidal ideation. I did not want to die! It was just me, Rob Pharazyn, versus some psychic, mythical force outside of me trying to convince me to move on from the planet, leave all the constant suffering behind and to go on to some better other life where peace and serenity prevailed. I often think that those that kill themselves are just seeking a 'break in the traffic', some silence, no static, no everything, and if they could get that, without total shutdown or death, then they would probably choose the option not to die by their own hand. My stronger self, Rob, would constantly tell the 'the force' whispering death in my mind to bugger off and leave me alone, whilst strange imagery would flash across my consciousness depicting a sort of paradise awaiting me if I only gave up the struggle.

One strong recurrent image that I do recall was of a beautiful, shiny black horse that was trapped and sinking in quicksand. The message that kept accompanying that image was 'don't struggle as you'll only sink further', which is very good advice in any dangerous situation.

I very much wanted to live but, I guess, my shadow self, ego and subconscious combo had a plan to convince me otherwise. Obviously, they lost because I'm still here! I resisted the force!

20

Narcotics Anonymous to the rescue

If you can imagine what it was like driving around the countryside, alone most of the time, half out of your mind with no one to talk to and only a large black, grinning poodle for company during the week, you'll probably start to get the picture of what my life was like at that time.

Every time I thought I'd sunk down to below my mental tolerance level in those dark days, there'd still be another trapdoor waiting there in the canyons of my mind, which would open up to take me down even further. Terrifying were those places in my mind where The Dark Shadow prowled around, whispering about death and madness, conspiring to kill me or drive me insane, whilst soaring above in the everyday innocent world, the seas were still deep blue, life went on and the sun shone down on the beautiful Byron Bay coastline.

When I had my next appointment, I told Jane the counsellor about my loneliness (never mention suicide to counsellors as they'll have you banged up in no time, supposedly for your own good) and she said to me that what I needed was some sort of structure to my days and suggested I meet up with Red, a local hard case and fully-fledged member of the Narcotics Anonymous (NA) chapters.

She gave me Brother Red's phone number and from that point on the game changed big-time as I tumbled down the rabbit hole into the parallel universe of addicts from all over Australia (but mainly the wild Kings Cross area of Sydney, Australia's biggest city) all trying to get clean by attending their nightly meetings of NA. That night, I rang Red and we arranged to meet.

Red, God bless him, was your typical suntanned Aussie hard case and a total character. He took me on like a fledgling duck that he'd found on the side of the road and away we went. He was a good-looking little bugger in a Jimmy Buffett sort of way and was into surfcast fishing from the beach, spinning yarns and knew everything that was going on up and down the coast.

His backstory was that he'd been an alcoholic and also a big-time coke user of gear, mainly from Asia. Having easy access to coke, he soon became a prodigious snorter of the 'marching powder' but, like all addicts, the time came when his drug of choice stopped working and as the saying goes, 'enough is never enough', so, combined with marital pressure, Red had come in from the cold and had joined the local Narcotics Anonymous with the intention of getting clean.

When I hooked up with him he'd been in their loop for quite a while and had passed his induction period. (I've read about getting tokens for days clean, but I think that's an American concept as I never saw any evidence of it.)

Like some secret society, NA and AA both like to keep their protocols under wraps, but I don't think it matters for me to talk about it here as my comments are all positive and what they offer, be it for booze or drug addiction withdrawal, is really the only available gateway out of madness during recovery from addiction and is an honest starting point on your walk back to sanity. I can't recommend it highly enough.

Having made the major breakthrough of Step One, which is admitting that you were powerless over your addiction (be it drugs or booze) and that your life had become unmanageable, one of the next protocols they like you to do upon joining is what they call '90 meetings in 90 days'. This requires a test of your level of commitment to get clean. There are nightly meetings scattered everywhere in any town, city or country around the world, but in this instance, you had to find a way to attend a meeting every night for 90 days somewhere across the Byron Bay region.

Given most boozers or junkies have hit rock bottom and don't have a car or even money for a bus, it's a fairly tall order, but they seem to do it, usually by car pooling, and I did my share of that down the track. A lot of the junkies, when I was deeper in amongst them, used to marvel at the fact that I actually had a car and a late-model one at that. Apparently, a rare commodity in the world of those who had fallen through the cracks in life and ended up at NA was to have a car.

Within a few days of bonding with my new-found mate, Red, the time came for me to take the next step. And so it came to pass on a balmy June evening that I ended up at my first meeting of Narcotics Anonymous with Brother Red. The assembled bunch of junkies were shuffling around outside the hall, puffing away on the only allowed addiction of roll-your-own cigarettes at this one of their many regular meeting places. In this instance, it was a local community hall at a laid-back town called Brunswick Heads, just north of Byron Bay and not far from South Golden Beach where I was living.

Byron Bay, to the uninitiated, is located on the east coast, just south of the Queensland border, and is the alternative, cosmic capital of Australia. The region has more freaks per square metre than anywhere else in the country, having been a big-time hippie Mecca in the seventies, and is also known as one of the most idyllic spots you could ever hope to find, with golden beaches and endless sunny days. (For American readers, think a mixture of Laurel Canyon with Carmel and Florida Keys.)

However, for the small band assembled on that night, there were no sunny days; just constant suffering as they tried their best to overcome years of savage drug addiction to everything from coke to heroin to all manner of other exotic but illegal drugs. As the tropical sun set over Mt Warning in the west, we filed into the hall to our hard, wooden seats and the meeting was opened with a greeting of welcome by what seemed to be the appointed 'convener' of the night, and this was then followed by a tilt to the death that day in Sydney from an overdose of 'smack' of well-known heroin user and top Australian painter, Brett Whiteley.

Bear in mind this was my first time to such a gathering, so

I was unprepared for the wailing and nodding that accompanied the news of Whiteley's death. As it rose to a chattering crescendo, a tall good-looking man resembling actor George Hamilton and wearing a cattleman's Driza-Bone full-length, oilskin overcoat leapt to his feet and started yelling and swearing about something completely unintelligible. Throwing back his coat it was apparent that maybe he had, what appeared to my eyes anyway, a sawn-off shotgun attached to the inside. Having heard Brother Red talking to him outside the hall and ascertaining that this guy was an ex-bank robber and coke dealer from Kings Cross in Sydney, made all his yelling resemble something out of a Tarantino movie, which was quite disturbing from where I was sitting, given my fragile and anxious drug-withdrawal newbie state of mind.

At that moment of graphic convergence, I truly felt like I really had stumbled down that metaphoric rabbit hole and a wave of deep despair washed over me, as it dramatically occurred to me that something had indeed gone very, very wrong with my life.

How did a well-educated, private boarding school boy from New Zealand take the wrong turns that had conspired to lead me to be surrounded by these obviously troubled flotsam and jetsam of life? A collection of battered souls who would normally be way out of my comfort zone and not the type of people I'd been used to hanging out with?

But what was normal any more?

The format of an NA (or Alcoholics Anonymous) meeting is the same all over the world. After the initial greetings and personal acknowledgements to familiar faces, the floor is opened for anyone who would like to 'share' whatever was on their mind. This meant that any addict at the meeting could volunteer to say, completely uncensored, anything he or she wanted, be it short or long in duration (and believe me, some of them were very long and rambling).

It involved the person recounting how they came to be at the meeting and what set of circumstances in their earlier life had brought them to that point. A typical opener would be 'Hi, my name is Billy and I'm an addict.' Then everyone would mumble 'Hi, Billy' and away Billy would go with his sad story about whatever he chose to talk about on that given night.

It was compulsory to have that opening line about being an addict, because if you couldn't or wouldn't admit you were an addict, then the credo was that you still weren't ready for recovery from your drug dependency and shouldn't be at the meeting. Although I never verbalised my thoughts and always went along with that opening line when it came to my turn to share ('Hi, my name is Rob and I'm an addict'), I personally never thought of myself as a junkie addict. You may ask what I mean by that.

Well, to me there is a subtle and sublime difference when coming to terms with addiction. In my mind, I was an 'accidental addict' through no fault of my own, due to being given prescription drugs without good advice.

Yes, I was an addict in recovery like everyone else at the meetings and I never resiled from that reality, but unlike my fellow desperates, who had ripped into all nature of drugs, recreationally, to get high or whatever, I never felt my daily intake of Ativan was in the same league.

I was right and I was wrong to some degree in my mental distinction because although virtually all the 'Na-Nas' at the meetings were hardcore drug users and thrillseekers we had one thing in common, which was whether it was prescription pills, like Ativan, or illegal drugs, like heroin, we had all been using the drugs to mask some internal mental pain or anxiety.

And therein lies the rub. Be it drugs, porn or alcohol, etc., they are all means of avoiding some buried pain trapped deep in your being, and until they are given recognition and attended to by being taken into the bright light of day at a meeting or maybe by trusted therapy, whatever your addiction is will continue to take you down, down, down until you either admit defeat and get yourself to a meeting, seek help of some kind, or die.

21

Brother Red and the Na-Na meetings

As I sat in my first meeting that night in Brunswick Heads with Brother Red, the first thing that struck me as different members, both male and female, went through the process of verbally sharing their tragic life stories, was the commonality of each story and even more scary was that I heard people admitting things that I thought were exclusive to me. It's a very strange feeling to hear a total stranger recount stories from his or her life, which was completely foreign to yours, and describing things that happened to him or her, that you thought applied to you only, hidden in the inner recesses of your mind and personal background.

So, the first reassuring thing about the infrastructure of NA is the fact that what you thought was your own private story of fears, failings and doubts was not just your burden alone and other people were suffering identical fears and doubts. It is very comforting to know that you're not alone in how you have viewed and experienced your perception of your previous life. To know others also went through the same reactions to life and addiction and were going through drug withdrawal as you were, gives you a sense of camaraderie, which is nourishing spiritually and engenders a feeling like you're coming in from the parched desert after you've been floundering around on your own throughout your life, prior to discovering NA.

Some addicts' 'shares' would get dark and brutal when people would, over future meetings I attended, disclose horrific stories of sexual abuse, theft, dishonesty, phony cons, scams and worse. Globally, drug addiction is the main driver of crime as addicts will steal, kill or do anything to get another hit, so pretty, young ex-prostitutes, bank robbers and violent criminals all attempting to become clean were at those meetings trying their level best to get away from lives of having to do anything to get money to feed their hopelessness and addiction. More power to them!

If I hadn't hooked up with Brother Red and moved into the world of the 'Na-Nas', I doubt whether I would be alive today and writing this book.

I'm not being overdramatic when I say that. In the meetings and the crew I hung out with over the coming months, I found a structure and purpose without which what was left of my flimsy soul, battered by self-detox and emotional withdrawal, would probably have eventually succumbed to the darkness calling from my shadow self and I would have taken my life.

Not because I wanted to die but because there is only so much mental torture you can process alone, without support, before you become way too lost to ever find your way out and, following the wrong star home, I would have gone.

As I said earlier, I always felt that I didn't really qualify in my benzo addiction to be a 'paid up' member of Narcotics Anonymous, but when talking to fellow members they'd often ask what my drug of 'choice' was and when I told them it was benzos, albeit not actually of my choosing, they would all, without exception, say that in the hardcore drug world, coming off benzodiazepines was recognised by junkies as being the hardest of all drugs to detox from.

Far worse than heroin apparently, as at least with heroin and other drugs you get methadone, etc. to help you down, but there is no chemical assistance when you detox from benzos, just ill-advised cold turkey or gradual withdrawal, so I was treated with respect by my fellow addicts, which again was important to my sense of being and place in the scheme of things.

Byron Bay, at that time, housed one of Australia's biggest 'boot camp' drug rehab centres, which was located on the edge of the town up on Binna Burra Road near Bangalow and was known as 'The Buttery'.

I never found out why it was called that because there were certainly no cows being milked up that end of town; only junkies from all over the country living there 24/7 for as long as it took to get clean and back into society. It's still successfully operating with a long waiting list due to it's reputation for turning people's lives around. I never went in there but the Buttery crew would be guaranteed to turn up to all the NA meetings. Their 'shares' or personal stories were always the most colourful and, once again, many times

I thought to myself, 'that could be my story' and that person sitting opposite me in the meeting could be me.

22

Was my life ruined by benzos?

They had a saying at NA that I have hung on to for a long time, which was 'You only get what you're ready for, never more than you can handle; and it does get better.' And this is how it turned out for me.

The human spirit or mind needs to have something to cling on to as you process your way out of withdrawal and this mantra served me well. The credo of Narcotics Anonymous was that the members all had a guardian angel or force greater than yourself that watched over you as you progressed through your recovery. It was often referred to as your 'HP', or 'higher power', and that saying that you never get more than you can handle, etc. was basically ascribed to the protection by your 'HP' over your wellbeing.

It was very comforting to believe that something greater than yourself was there for you. A lot will scoff at that, but don't knock it until you've been to the bottom of your life and tried working your way out again. If believing in a higher power or a guardian angel gets you through the mad days and dark nights, then that was good enough for me! Where I was at, I would've believed in a blunt screwdriver if I thought it was going to relieve my suffering!

Anyone coming off benzos (or other drugs) and reading my story may be wondering by now how or why would I get myself hooked up with a bunch of crazies and criminals with a reliance on higher powers when all I wanted to do was to get through my drug withdrawal process and be free from pills? Why didn't I throw myself at the mercy of the medical system and government agencies in the outside world?

Ha! That's what got me into trouble in the first place. I've read recently published books by others who have tried withdrawing from benzos via the mainstream conventional systems, such as psychiatrists and rehab units, and have ended up worse off or back on some sort of meds for the rest of their long, lonely lives. Give me the assorted and divinely flawed critters of NA any day over that other option. Based on experience, my very best advice to you is that being with damaged but non-judgmental people who all had something in common and understood the withdrawal process such as my fellow 'Na-Nas' could offer, is preferable to what the conventional world and supposed medical professionals can ever put forward as a solution.

As I indicated in the beginning of my story, there aren't many books out there which can give you a blow-by-blow map as to how to survive and get through the first year of absolute torture and subsequent recovery trauma.

Despite intense Googling, I've only managed to find maybe 10 personally written accounts available on Amazon and other online booksellers, of individuals actually 'walking the walk' and overcoming the benzo devil.

Benzo addiction and the withdrawal process has become a large bandwagon due to the huge problem that it is and a lot people are jumping on it to try to make a buck. There are plenty of books written by psychiatrists, scientists and new age authors giving screeds of scientific and probably helpful general information, but these books are based on clinical observation. Given benzos are still being prescribed by the millions every day, it seems those books are essentially superfluous in making any difference, other than supplying heaps of semi-scientific or garbled information which would conceivably only serve to confuse an actual addict looking for a way out of addiction. It's not rocket science. You're an addict, you're trapped, you want to know how to get out! Keep it simple but factual.

Those few books on addiction and recovery, which I've sourced globally, have mainly been written by Americans and all recount horrific misadventures suffered by those in withdrawal at the hands of doctors and psychiatrists.

I bought one book off Amazon which was basically a well-intentioned horror story written by a woman relating her unfortunate experiences with multiple brands of benzo drugs of fairly high dosages.

On the very first page of the book, she recounts her early attempt at withdrawal which led her to jumping off a local bridge in a suicide attempt. This poor woman subsequently (according to her book) ended up having holes drilled in her skull under medical supervision and apparently suffering more clinical travesties by psychiatrists during attempted withdrawal and with no seemingly apparent satisfactory ending. Fortunately, at the end of the story, her Christian faith was fulfilling her nowadays as she avoided self-pity and answers to the burning questions of 'Why me?' and 'What did I do to deserve having my life ruined by benzos?' I genuinely wish her good fortune because at least she tried. But where's the inspiration to get off the pills if all your story can tell the world is that your life ended up still being miserable?

To my mind, there has got to be an incentive towards a brighter, new world of clarity to encourage addicts to rid themselves of their addiction. I wouldn't be writing this book if all I could offer you was my story of going through abject hell, only to eventually end up drug-free but on a welfare benefit in a rental bedsit somewhere in the boondocks, staring at the next door neighbour's tin fence.

Most of you reading this book already know that you're caught up in a horror movie called 'your addiction', so why pay to read about frightening stuff unless there is a chance of a hopeful outcome? There's little point in reading something that just reaffirms that you're stuck in an addictive nightmare.

Therefore, I'm writing this book to offer you a voice of experience, as someone who has walked that walk (and I certainly have done that) and can offer you practical steps to recovery and proof that a great life after addiction can be achieved if you will only just take that first step.

Seeking help from most doctors to get off benzos is generally of no use as they have little interest or, for that matter, any knowledge about addiction withdrawal. The question would have to be, if they knew about the horrors of withdrawal, why would they prescribe benzos ongoing to patients in the first place?

Surely, they wouldn't be so irresponsible? Or would they? Having said that, I think it's worth searching around the region where you live and try to find a medical professional who is more holistic in their approach to patient care, and then quiz them on their knowledge of benzodiazepine withdrawal. But take care not to be blinded by the 'doctor knows best' syndrome. What you're looking for is 'managed wellness' of your own health and you must take control of that process, so keep looking till you find a sympathetic doctor before you make the biggest decision of your life to enter self-detox and discontinuation.

23

Nimbin, pythons and synchronicity

As in all nightmares, there is usually a break in the traffic and some respite, albeit only brief. This came for me in the form of hooking up with another new Na-Na friend, called Axel, so now not only did I have Brother Red to sit around in the sun swapping hard luck stories with, I also had Axel, who was a whole new bowl of toenail clippings. He was in his late twenties, highly intelligent, and in a previous life had been an IT expert for the Australian government.

Unfortunately, he had found 'chasing the dragon' of heroin to be more fun than writing software programs and had soon become addicted to hard drugs. He was what we called a 'drug warrior'.

Some people can handle powerful drugs and some can't. Axel was one of the former and his idea of fun on a Saturday night had been to pop an LSD trip under each eyelid so the 'acid' hit the 'high speed' (excuse the pun) button and went straight to the brain, swallow a couple of Ecstasy pills backed up with a strong joint of weed, a taste of smack and then head out for a night's fun!

He'd ended up living in the hills behind Byron at the very well-known stoner town of Nimbin, which is where the real hard-core, latter-day hippies and flower children had gravitated to since the seventies post-Woodstock era.

The dream had started off well with their Aquarius Festival in 1973, drawing in the 'hips' by the thousands, but, unfortunately, over the years, the peace, love and flowers groove had all but gone and Nimbin had pretty much become a rather tragic drug haven. Some very good dope was grown there and it was common knowledge that wherever you lived around the coast, Nimbin was the place to go for an easy, guaranteed score. An annual event that attracted thousands was the MardiGrass, which kept the local cops busy as the hippies drove through the main street of Nimbin on the back of a flatbed truck, throwing out hundreds of pre-rolled joints to the grateful crowd, who were all as high as kites in the carnival atmosphere.

However, in the late eighties, the ravages of heroin had arrived in Nimbin and around 11am most mornings, the Israeli and German 'smack' dealers would glide into town in their silver Mercedes.

The locals would be cashed up from selling weed around the cafes earlier in the morning and would then buy their bags of powder and so the day would go around. Axel was very much part of that loop and was also, apparently, a very skilled artisan and award-winning grower of weed.

Like most junkies, he and his girlfriend were both into heroin as their drug of choice, so it took a lot of courage for him to leave her behind and come down from the hills to start going to meetings to get clean.

One day, Axel asked me if I could drive him back up to Nimbin to get his guitar and belongings from where he and his girlfriend had been living, and as I was the only person in the Na-Na tribe with a car, I happily agreed. It was an extremely hot Saturday afternoon as we drove into Nimbin, with hippies popping their heads up like meerkats from their various psychedelic shacks to check us out as we sailed on by. We got to his girlfriend's hangout and there was no one there, so we wandered around looking inside for Axel's belongings. I totally freaked out when I walked into the bathroom and there was a very large, colourful python curled up around the base of the toilet bowl. Apparently, in the hot, dry Australian weather, snakes come inside looking for water. Fortunately, the tree pythons are harmless, but I didn't hang round to find out. (Maybe his girlfriend had been a stripper, as they had a habit of keeping pet pythons.)

By now, Axel had ascertained that his guitar and stuff were gone, so we spun up to some hippie's place that he knew. Next minute, there's yelling and banging, with clothes and a guitar flying out a side window and then an extremely agitated Axel returned, dumped everything in my car and said, 'Let's go!' It turned out that the ex-girlfriend had sold most of his other stuff to this hippie so she could buy more drugs. The guitar he'd thrown into my car was not actually Axel's, but who cares? 'Vengeance is mine', sayeth the angry junkie (and the Lord), and as bushranger Ned Kelly said on the gallows, 'Such is life!'

It was a dangerous emotional event for Axel to undertake, going back on that day, as the sheer heartache of his girlfriend shacking up with another junkie and ripping off his gear would've been a likely trigger for him to buckle under the strain and 'pick up' the dope again, but he didn't.

Everything in life is tribal, even at NA meetings, and you soon found people who would gravitate towards you for a variety of reasons, allowing you to find your own level of friends and make up a cohort of like minds. Axel was a real tonic for me, as he was funny and intelligent so we soon became good mates.

I was still living up the coast at South Golden Beach and trying to get to as many meetings as possible, as they were the only place I felt some sense of structure in my state of mind, but the distance down to Byron and back was getting a bit tedious and expensive. I won't bore you with more sad tales of high anxiety and hallucinations, although some were quite interesting, if for no other reason than showing how the brain plays tricks on your perceptions. I can remember one night driving down to Byron for a meeting when all of a sudden, the road signs seemed to change into what looked like white horses charging towards me. Although only brief, it was still enough to keep me arced up to a fascinated but high-tension level.

And so the 'Na-Na' life became my everyday scene. By day, Axel and I would hang around the parks with the other desperates, talking bullshit or aimlessly wandering the beaches outlining our dreams and schemes for the future if it ever arrived, and then by night we'd go to meetings. They'd be in different areas around the region and most nights we'd find ourselves, as usual, sitting around in cold community halls listening to all the forlorn tales of the newbies who'd drifted in. Sometimes guest speakers would turn up driving flash cars, to tell us all about how they'd become clean after years of drug use and then gone on to lead miraculous lives and we'd all mumble 'Yeah, right' under our breath. Some were on the level, but you can't fool the junkies and it was common knowledge that a few amongst this so-called 'drug royalty' were maybe no longer using dope themselves, but were now dealing dope, which has to be the lowest of the low. Talk about identifying your target customer base.

They say that life is just six degrees of separation between all of us, and this was demonstrated to me one particular night when I was at a meeting at Bangalow, on the outskirts of Byron.

It was a full crew and as I looked around the room, I spotted a familiar face from way back in my past. After the meeting came to a close and the usual Serenity prayer ('God, grant me the serenity to accept the things I cannot change, the courage to change the things I can, and the wisdom to know the difference') had been said as we all held hands in a circle, the familiar face wandered over and greeted me by a nickname which I'd had as a kid at boarding school in New Zealand. I knew him quite well back at college, although he'd been expelled from school for so-called 'daring practices', so it was fascinating to hear his tale of how his life had played out since getting 'the boot'.

A bad speed and heroin habit, Thailand and all kinds of drug dens in South-East Asia had ruled his life and now the cosmos had conspired under the weird laws of synchronicity to bring our paths together, once again, after nearly 30 years. Like me, he'd also come from a well-off, New Zealand family background. Now, most of his teeth were missing from heroin usage, he looked about 80 years old but good on him; he was obviously trying to get clean. We had a bit of a chat about life in general and then we joined the last of the Na-Nas melting away from the meeting and into the night. I stopped for a while and chatted to Dove, the sax player who had had a big-name career as a session muso in the States, backing bands like the Eagles and releasing his own albums. Lovely fellow! Apparently, he went on to make successful music both in Australia and New York. Sadly, he died in 2016 of cancer.

The last time I ever saw my old boarding school friend was a few months later. He was standing on a street corner outside the Byron Bay hospital holding a small, battered brown suitcase, looking very alone. He told me he was off to try to make it in the outside world and I've often wondered how he got on. Most likely dead!

There's a humorous saying in the NA and AA world that says when you go to the meetings and get yourself well, your life becomes like a cowboy song in reverse. You get your horse back, your girlfriend, your home and the bank loves you again! In truth, a lot of junkies find it just too hard out there in the abnormal world and lapse back and never, ever get close to that cowboy song. This is where the concept of having a personal sponsor kicks in. A sponsor is someone who has stayed 'clean' for a lengthy period who can team up with you to be your 24/7 wingman, so if you feel emotionally or physically incapable of staying away from drugs or alcohol, then they're there for you night and day to talk you through any mini-crisis and hopefully prevent you from lapsing (or 'picking up', as it's known in NA jargon).

Sponsors are a very good idea and should be considered by anyone in early recovery. I didn't bother initiating a spon-

sor because at an intellectual and co-dependency level, I
didn't feel the need, although I was still very much struggling
in my own world of recovery and withdrawal.

I'd had a bad experience with my counsellor, Jane, at the
Mullumbimby Hospital Drug and Alcohol unit, which had
caused me to cut her loose from the slipstream of my life in
the interests of self-preservation as I saw it at the time.

She'd done her best over the previous few months and
had pointed me in the direction of Brother Red and NA, but
she had now concluded in our weekly meetings that I wasn't
improving quickly enough and indicated that I should seriously consider going into a Salvation Army rehab unit for a
while, to get the support she considered that I needed.

I'm sure she had the best of intentions, but this really
freaked me out, so I figured that I was starting to again be
relegated to the 'one size fits all, plan B' model for struggling addicts, rather than the personal, one-on-one input I'd
had from her so far. So I decided I didn't need her advice
to do an Amy Winehouse, even though it was probably well
meant. (It's important you follow your instincts in recovery,
as one misstep with the system and you can end up lost all
over again.)

After the meeting with her, I went back to where I was
staying at the beach and, in a confused and agitated flurry
of tears, told Frank about her proposal. Good ol' Frank
responded by saying, 'Over my dead body will that happen.'
That's what friends are about. Frank died recently, after a
good innings, and he was one of the genuine but flawed
members of the cosmic cowboys, all struggling to be free.

I kept in touch with Jane occasionally after that and I'm
sure she would've been there for me if I'd needed her input,

which turned out to be correct when I tried to claim compensation in New Zealand for medical misadventure. But, we'll get to that later!

24

Time to move forward on the quest

Hopefully, by now you will have gathered from my story so far that to try to withdraw from benzos and go into recovery alone is just simply not advisable. You need some sort of structure around you; and well-meaning professionals, like the Salvation Army or doctors, don't cut it. You're better off amongst people who have 'walked the walk', which is again why I strongly advocate doing what I did, which was to immerse myself into that non-judgmental and friendly NA culture. The outside perception of the types of people who become junkies and go to Narcotics Anonymous meetings is wrong. You can't possibly judge unless you've been there and attended meetings.

Some were definitely not to be trusted, but most were just damaged individuals who'd made a series of bad choices or had had a terrible time as children with sexual abuse, cruel or criminal parents, etc. There's research that shows

48% of all alcoholics and drug addicts are self-medicating to dampen down the internal pain, anxiety, depression, whatever, but they're not all hooked on dope or booze just for partying and fun reasons.

It's tempting to keep writing about all the weird and often quirky anecdotes that happened during my days with the Na-Nas, because they were very fascinating times and rather like living on another planet. However, I knew deep down that if I didn't break myself out of the downward spiral and semi-feral lifestyle that I was living, I would never get out of there and that would be it. Long hair, leather hat and a wooden, walking wizard pole for Rob as he impersonated being a freak and an ageing hippy. No way! There was a better life out there somewhere in the gloom and I had to find it. Plus, there was every chance that if I didn't try to keep moving, I could end up taking benzos again or worse, as most days I really could see no future for myself. Not in my wildest dreams could I have imagined how it actually did turn out.

I was once caught in a bad rip off the beach at Surfers Paradise on the Gold Coast and as I struggled in the panic to get out of the ocean's pull, I could see life going on as normal, with cars zipping down the coastal highway and people playing on the beach while I was going under, and that was very much how I felt in my current situation. The modern world sped on past me each day as I trudged along at turtle speed trying to rewire my mind and figure out which way was the best way out.

I decided that it was also time to get out of the comfort zone at Frank and Ava's. Things had started to get weird when a fat Greek man moved into the luxury beach house next door and told Frank that he was a novelist writing Western novels, so he liked his privacy and often worked through the night. Frank, being a very straight guy whose only vice was the bottle, believed him, but in a short space of time the obviously wasted-looking young girls staggering around the beach and the black SUVs coming and going in the dead of night alerted my knowing brain to the fact that there was more than cowboys and Indians going on next door. Easy answer was to ask around at the next NA meeting and sure enough, our new neighbour was a big-time heroin dealer who had arrived up from the glitter of Sydney to set up shop. It didn't take long before I was awoken at dawn with the sounds of a full-scale police bust going down next door and that was the end of our local Western novelist. They were all gone in around 60 seconds in the back of a patrol car without so much as a wave goodbye.

For weeks after that, you'd see shadowy figures skulking around the garden and sand hills at night with torches weaving about, as the rumour had got around the dope scene that the bust had been so quick that Greek Costa hadn't had time to uplift his hidden stash of heroin. So the dopers were now trying to find it in the garden and sand dunes, apparently without success, although urban legend had it that it was a large stash and was definitely still there, hidden in the shifting, whispering sands.

In my endeavours to move on, I answered an advertisement in the local newspaper, *The Echo*, and soon found myself sharing a house in Coorabell, overlooking Byron Bay, with three Germans. The landlord was well-known, offbeat English violinist Nigel Kennedy. One of the Germans, Helmut, was a former sannyasin, or Osho Orange religion follower, and was as nutty as a fruitcake. He told me that his father had disowned him back in Germany, but that was fine by him. He said he could understand his father not liking him because 900 years earlier his father had been a female concubine in Helmut's harem when he was an Arabian king and he had treated his father/mother badly, so his karma was to be disowned in this present life for his past kingly bad behaviour.

The other couple of Germans, Arki and Lukas, had gone through sham marriages to try to get Australian residency and were very pleasant and totally straight. They were constantly being turned over by the male and female Australians that they had entered into the shams with and the sneaky Aussies would forever be ringing up needing more money or to be taken out to lavish meals on the premise that Immigration had been hanging around and they all needed to get their stories on the same page. I felt sorry for the two serious Germans and I heard many years later that they broke up as a couple.

On my part, it was and it wasn't a good idea to make the move to start sharing with total strangers of a foreign nationality. It would be anxiety-inducing enough for anyone under normal circumstances, but for me it was a bit of a high-wire act, as they had no idea about my life or Ativan addiction recovery scene and probably just thought I was a nice New Zealand guy who seemed a bit odd. I spent a lot of my time hiding in my magnificent bedroom overlooking a vast expanse of coastal ocean feeling threatened by almost everything, including a kangaroo that used to lurk in the garden nearby.

25

Giving something back

You may think by now that my physical withdrawal symptoms would have passed and to a large degree they had, other than the ongoing chronic insomnia and constant high anxiety.

The earlier racking symptoms of blinding headaches, nerve spasms and pain had dissipated to a bearable degree, but the ongoing ride of months and grinding months of withdrawal stage two, the emotional detox, was still really challenging me.

The problems had always been there in the past, ticking away at a muted level back in the days of taking the benzos, but, like the sound of a train coming from a long way off, it got louder and louder as the days and months after ceasing taking Ativan rolled on by and the lid continued to really fly off my internal rubbish tin.

Just when you think that you must've seen all the crap

inside your mind since the emotional withdrawal episodes had kicked in months earlier after the physical side had calmed down slightly, another barrage of jumbled pictures from the past comes knocking, demanding attention (and I mean really demanding!). Deep, acute, mental loneliness, the ongoing constant suicidal ideation, sleep deprivation, heightened nightmares. They were all there like a daily chorus hounding me with a vengeance.

Everything I'd known to be me throughout my life was being challenged by my psyche, bringing on a sense of loss of personal identity, paranoia and fear. Imagine having to relive all the past hurts, fears and misguided thinking of your life all over again, as the mental filing system tries to process everything in an attempt to refile the updated thoughts into my new, non-benzo dependent brain. Like a computer server gone mad, they were now downloading random stuff into my consciousness at a furious pace. This montage of madness, mayhem and my past were my constant companions, riding shotgun along beside and inside me like the Grim Reaper in my daily existence. My mind felt like mud and seemed to work incredibly slowly as I desperately tried putting together viable concepts for my daily survival. Talk about cognitive dissonance.

What a bloody nightmare but I survived it!

I think the deep feeling of complete, abject hopelessness for my future was the worst. I could see no way that I could ever get back to a decent, balanced level of life, if for no other reason than that I couldn't envisage getting my mind together enough to be able, in any way, to generate an income to get free from the trap which I was in.

Ironically, a few years earlier I'd acquired full Australian citizenship which gave me a dual nationality passport for both New Zealand and Australia and, at the time I acquired it, I'd thought in the back of my mind that at least Australia was warm, so if I ended up on the bones of my arse living as a 'parrothead' in a trailer park somewhere sunny, north of the Tropic of Capricorn, shelling tiger prawns and drinking rum as I faded into total mediocrity, then things could be a lot worse. Little did I know those few years back, just how close to reality things were now beginning to shape up for my future.

As a rule, humans tend to predominantly focus, when in survival mode, on threats or negative stimuli. This response is controlled by two almond-shaped neurons known as the amygdala, which is located deep in the brain's medial temporal lobe, near the hippocampus which is inside the skull from the ear. In humans and other animals, this subcortical brain structure is linked to both the fear and pleasure responses and is responsible for bringing us all our daily stress and anxiety if it's not correctly balanced. This gland has been with us since the caveman days and controls our 'fight or flight' response by pumping floods of cortisol and adrenaline into our system and shutting down peripheral faculties when we feel under threat of any sort. (Try jamming on your brakes when a car appears out of nowhere and you'll feel these reactions very clearly.)

Modern research has found that while most people automatically tend towards negative stimuli and seem to find it easier to be unhappy than happy, given the proper ability and motivation they can show the same response but in the positive, not in the 'fight or flight' mode, by giving gestures of kindness.

Scientists have found that the amygdala, which drives all your anxious thinking, may also be at the heart of compassion. Researchers have scanned participants' brains while they viewed pictures of people that were in need of either help or compassion. The data they saw clearly indicated that amygdala activity spiked when participants observed people in need, which was particularly true for those who scored high in empathy.

From this research I had stumbled upon, I picked up on the possibility of some peace of mind. So chasing a calmer amygdala by giving out compassion instead of empty self-obsession, plus hoping for a further sense of structure in my life, I volunteered at the local community Neighbourhood Centre in Mullumbimby, near Byron town, in an attempt to give myself a better sense of purpose. (I know. It's a very long-winded way to explain how to get that sense of purpose.)

Two afternoons a week, you'd find me talking to desperately poor people, handing out food parcels and money vouchers to keep them afloat. Unbeknownst to the unfortunates, like the duck on the lake surface, I was also paddling as fast as I could just to stay upright. Some of the people that came in were ones that I'd seen at Na-Na meetings but, similar to the Mafia Omerta code of silence, we didn't show any signs of recognition for each other.

In amongst sorting out paying electricity bills for the down-and-outs and handing out vouchers for much-needed clothes or furniture, there was a very pretty young woman in her late teens that used to come in regularly for food parcels and vouchers; then one day she stopped coming.

A week later they found her dead in a nearby creek with

her wrists slashed in an apparent suicide. I asked around and it seemed she was bipolar and, ironically, also coming off prescription meds and recreational drugs. She had found the going too tough and had gone back and taken the prescription meds, only to find they didn't work any more, so in the terror of ending up in a chemical no-man's-land, she'd killed herself.

It's hard to imagine what sort of hell she was in, with the last moments of her life bleeding away beside a muddy creek, far from home and no mother in sight. Tragic!

This is something to be very aware of when you start down the path of freedom from drugs.

There's the old saying around NA and AA that says, 'One is too many and a thousand is never enough', which appertains to what happens when considering hitting the bottle or the needle again. This also applies in reverse with chemical drugs from coke to benzos in that if you withdraw for a period of time and then try to go back, you'll most likely find that you get no response or high like you'd been used to in the past.

Only panic, a scrambled brain and crippling fear all over you.

Many benzodiazepine users who find themselves in this position have withdrawn too quickly or have made the foolish decision and gone 'cold turkey'. Finding the going too tough after months of withdrawal, they think that if they go back to again taking benzodiazepines (aw, just a few won't hurt?), they will be more successful next time they decide to try to give up the pills. Unfortunately, it doesn't seem to work that way. For reasons that are not clear, but perhaps because the original experience of withdrawal has already sensitised the nervous system and heightened the level of anxiety, the original benzodiazepine dose often doesn't work the second time round. There's probably always exceptions, but can you imagine the panic you would feel if you went back, only to find that the drugs had no effect any more? It would be better to press on with withdrawal than face that nightmare.

I simply cannot emphasise this enough and it's crucial that you absorb it before you start out. You can slow down your initial speed of shaving down the pills in early withdrawal and reset the daily amount, but once you've been 'clean' for a month or two, there should be no thoughts of going back as you set sail on the voyage of discovering your new, clean and shiny self!

I also repeat from earlier in this book that when you first get down to taking no more prescription meds and becoming drug-free after having had a long period of artificially supplying your brain chemistry with a pill, your brain has long ago ceased producing the natural anxiety-reducing chemicals to attach to your GABA receptors as it's designed to do from the day you were born. Consequently, when you enter the initial protracted withdrawal and you're no longer swallowing a daily pill of artificial GABA, your nervous system, mind and drug-free brain are now living in a very scary twilight world where a piece of paper blowing down the street can induce a panic attack.

The rule of thumb is that your anxiety levels in the early withdrawal stages and for a while in the ensuing totally drug-free months are, according to research, magnified by up to 13 times higher than what they would be expected to be as a normal reaction to an everyday situation, so life can get pretty scary in the early self-detox, withdrawal days. The good news is that it does pass and it does slowly settle down — all you have to do is 'ride the storm' until the peace of mind cavalry start to show up.

Breathe, just breathe.

This is very common advice but in these circumstances, it could be the difference between winning and losing.

26

Taking that next big step

I carried on beavering along at the Neighbourhood Community Centre in Mullum and found it to be quite rewarding and would suggest that anyone in recovery gives some worthwhile volunteer work a shot. However, it personally took me all my mental reserves to decipher a multitude of normal events that presented themselves daily, without my freaking out and losing it.

Of course, social anxiety and agoraphobia come with the territory in recovery and these two factors are often the original reasons why a lot of socially shy people resort to script drugs in the first place. But you must resist the urge to panic when confronted by something that appears confusing, as it's totally not necessary to get flustered. Whatever is in front of your eyes and in your mixed-up brain that appears to be insurmountable and scary, is quite easily resolved and would be what everyday people would call a normal situation that most contend with as they go about their daily grind.

Fear thrives on resistance so the more your try to dampen it down the more it comes on. A trick that always worked well for me was to mentally look at the fear building inside you and say *"C'mon fear. Give me ya best shot...bring it on!"* and then imagine this cloud of fear floating over your *left* shoulder and disappearing. Believe me. It does work.

It seems a vicious but not unbeatable circle, if you hold steady and take your time to try to rationally process your thoughts throughout your given day. There is absolutely no hurry to be right or resolve anything, as you're not going anywhere in the outside world until you get well again, so just take it one day or one minute at a time, as the song says. It's no big deal! There aren't any. And always remember that the person in front of you can't see inside your head, so if you remain calm, they'll never know the difference.

Having finally reached the night-time at the end of each day, I would fall exhausted into a broken sleep and then have to contend with nightmares, night sweats, etc. only to wake in the morning, full of anxiety at the thought of having to start at the bottom of the mountain and climb up to the end of another day all over again. I don't think that feeling each morning has ever entirely gone away, so maybe that's just part of the price to pay.

There's no point in my belabouring the constant mental suffering I was going through, as it serves no useful purpose, but suffice to say most of my days were a continual struggle and just plain sad.

Fortunately, I'd now befriended a lovely woman who also worked at the Neighbourhood Centre in Mullum. Margie was part Aboriginal. She had been married to a man, now deceased, who had been wrongly convicted of murder prior to her meeting him but she had loved him all the same. She was one of the most kind-hearted people I had ever met and took me under her wing like a mother hen, cooking huge dinners, doing my washing and including me in her small family circle. She lived on her own in a big, old Queenslander house in Mullumbimby which had wide verandahs and was built high off the ground for air-flow purposes in the heat and to keep the snakes away over summer. In a short space of time she had invited me to move into one of the many rooms at her house, but with no romantic strings attached. This suited me as the Germans had become too complex to continue living with. By day they were a very dour bunch and set in their thinking, but by night, after a few handles of beer, they'd be yelling and playing loud oom-pah music as they catapulted off the walls, so it was time for me to go on to my next 'island'.

Margie and I hung out together like two little birds in the eye of the storm, as she was also a bit of an outsider through no fault of her own.

We roamed the backblock roads of northern New South Wales, by car, on sunny afternoons, eating carrot cake with coffees at places like the Crystal Castle, set high up in the hinterlands, and for the first time in many moons, her kind companionship gave me a modicum of sanity and peace around the edges of my fractured psyche. Maybe there was hope after all?

She could sense that I was going through something intense, but she wasn't the type to put her nose into my private life, so I told her that I was suffering from PTSD (post-traumatic stress disorder) after witnessing a shotgun murder back in New Zealand and she seemed content with that. My biggest curse of insomnia would see me many a time sitting in the dark early hours of the morning out on the verandah at her place in the humid Australian nights listening to the crickets chirping away and watching the strings of lightning arcing across the mountains as I tried to get my brain processes together enough to work out how to get myself back to normality. But what was that normality and what did it even look like now, after having had my brains fried?

The problem with insomnia, as many of you will know, is that it saps all your energy and robs you of the rational thought processes required to make quality decisions, so for me it was a bit like a salmon trying to swim up the rapids in a forlorn hope of reaching the spawning grounds, only to either get eaten by the bears on the river bank or flop around totally exhausted and no closer to my intended destination. How could I go forward when I didn't really know which way I was facing?

Because of the tenuous nature of my relationship with my family back in New Zealand (especially my mother), I'd felt very much like an exile in Australia during the recovery process. My constant fear of taking my life was starting to really swamp me, so I figured that if I was going to die it would be better to do it in my home country where at least I would get a decent burial, as opposed to shuffling off the planet in Byron Bay, where most of my current crop of 'friends', except for Margie, Frank and Ava, were addicts and misfits who were quite accustomed to paying homage at the nightly meetings to a fallen junkie who had found it all just too much to bear. A quick prayer and a nodding of heads was the most I could've expected from my troubled brethren, the Na-Nas.

Then things came to a head very quickly.

One dark, stormy night, like Heathcliff out of *Wuthering Heights*, I found myself wandering alone in a highly distressed state, on a beach at Belongil on the edge of Byron town, with the tears streaming down my face and yelling like a man possessed at the blustering winds and the gods. I can remember falling to my knees, arms raised to the sky and informing Mr God that I'd had enough, I was stuffed, couldn't take any more, and to strike me down there and then or bloody well help me! Nothing happened, but as the skies opened up and the thick droplets of rain started pelting down on my face, I felt a faint sense of something resembling hope shifting deep within me, with the inner message being for me to move on. (The crack in the sky is where the light comes in, maybe? Thanks, Leonard.)

The next day I hooked up with my mates, Axel and Brother Red, and told them that as far as I was concerned I had had an epiphany the night before that said that an endless round of NA meetings was just another form of addiction and that I was going to step off the carousel and head back to my home country. They both understood, although I could tell they had formed a substitute co-dependency on the weekly meetings so to them, the thought of 'going over the wall' seemed a very bold move. But the time had come for me to bid farewell to the Na-Nas and all the emotional sustenance they had provided me with during my darkest of dark days over the previous months.

I also came to realise after sitting through all the tortured recounting of personal stories by those addicts at the NA meetings that, in a sense, they were maybe addicted to not only drugs in their past, but addicted also to feeling constantly worthless as a way of defining themselves and that was not my issue. In fact, it was very much to the contrary.

It was now time to start the rebuild of my life and self-esteem and step number one was the Herculean task (or so it seemed) of getting myself back to New Zealand. All it involved was booking an airline ticket and working out the process of what to do with my car and meagre belongings, but the mere thought of dealing with the everyday world in a straight line, after nearly 12 months of living 'off the grid' in withdrawal, sent me into a total spin. My poor old cerebral cortex was still slaving away trying to repair the damaged neural pathways and I was by no means confident to do anything that required me to deal with the decision-making processes such as booking flight tickets, etc.

I rang my mother in New Zealand, told her that I was in dire straits (and I don't mean the band) and needed help, but in her usual form, she didn't offer much sympathy. However, it was getting near to Christmas by this time, so I said it'd be good to come home for a week or two over Christmas and she begrudgingly agreed. This solved my pathetic dilemma about the supposed enormity of my making the total move back home all in one hit. To relieve the pressure, my logic was to do it in two bites, and so it proved to be.

27

Family ... what family?

I left my car at my friend Margie's and flew home. I had been away for nearly five years, so it was easy to have fantasies, having been under the amount of pressure that I had suffered for so long.

I'd naïvely conjured up this image of being welcomed home like the proverbial, biblical prodigal son with the killing of the fatted calf and a big, happy feast, but that's not the way it worked out. (Like Danny in the hit Netflix TV series 'Bloodline', I wasn't at all well received.)

Even though they knew from my older brother who had flown over to Australia when I hit the wall earlier in withdrawal that I had been in serious emotional trouble, my family treated me as if my suffering over the past year was just some overly dramatic story that I'd cooked up to get sympathy. I can recall my younger brother saying to me that 'surely you can't expect us to believe that one little white pill could cause so much trouble for you' in a tone that indicated that there wasn't much understanding. However, he drove me around the countryside and the feeling of being in familiar surrounds again gave me enough much-needed direction to see a way forward.

I had become so staunch from my time at NA in Australia that I wouldn't take anything possibly addictive, right down to the manic level of things such as a Panadol or Coca-Cola, so I politely refused to have a drink with my family, which only served to make them less cordial.

It always amuses me when people crank on about the supposed bonds of family because it's invariably bullshit when the whip comes down and reality bites. In my opinion, it is often just a cliché that people mutter to delude themselves that they do care until confronted by a genuine family crisis, and then any meagre help offered is just to make them feel better about their emotionally bereft lives. You would've thought that my family would have wrapped around me to give me some sense of nurture and comfort, but it doesn't work like that in the dysfunctional orbit of a huge amount of families out there in the modern world.

I discovered that my mother had told her friends that I was home from Australia after having suffered a nervous breakdown, which, in a weird but unkind way, wasn't too far from the truth. However, nervous breakdowns happen to people who can't cope with their everyday lives, and overload. I think it would be fair to say that I had handled more pressure and stress in the last year than most people could bear in a lifetime and I was still functioning, albeit a little shaky. Nervous breakdowns didn't remotely relate in any way to the actual reality of my struggle with addiction withdrawal. Totally different department, but given they didn't really believe me when I told them the truth of what I'd been through and that the real me was still in complete control of my faculties underneath the burden I was coping with, it was an exercise in futility to try to haul some kindness from them into the equation and I couldn't do much more than wonder why a mother would do that to an obviously struggling son.

Psychologists subscribe to a popularly held belief that in dysfunctional families, the concept of a family member falling on hard times mentally (or suiciding) apparently allows the other family members to psychologically bundle up a collective-consciousness transference of their own past guilts and mental fears, which they then subliminally project onto the unfortunate, struggling family member. When that 'scapegoat' ends up being committed to an institution or dead, the other members of the dysfunctional family feel a sublime sense of exoneration and release from their own dark thoughts and misdeeds, as if the suicided family member has taken all the collective family dysfunction to the next world and those remaining feel a burden being lifted from their own miserable lives.

Not very pleasant, but apparently true, according to the shrink fraternity. Perhaps, after my being a dominant, alpha member of the family in the past, they felt their time had come to give me a good kicking and see me squirm, but they got that wrong.

I've given some serious thought as to whether I should include my personal family situation in this book, but the treatment I got was just part of a long history going right back to my childhood, which possibly led me to taking Ativan in the first place for anxiety reasons, and I suspect that some of you will recognise similar behaviour and dysfunction within your own family. I never really forgave my mother for those days, but she's no longer here so that's not an issue.

The upside of this family behaviour was that it offended and hurt me so deeply that it made me formulate the structure for a plan to continue my upward quest back to a worthwhile and benzo-free life. I decided that I would return to Byron Bay to bid farewell to my surrogate home of the last year and relocate back to New Zealand indefinitely. I'd cajoled my mother into agreeing to allow me to stay at the family home until I got things sorted, knowing full well that this would really motivate me to 'bite the bullet' and get moving towards finding work, my own place and, hopefully, some semblance of a new life. I flew back to Australia, sold my car and said goodbye to that chapter of my withdrawal and slow recovery from the devil benzodiazepine prescription drug, Ativan.

It really did seem like I'd come from another planet back to a nasty reality being in New Zealand full time again. Although the previous year in Brisbane and Byron where I'd taken those first steps into withdrawal had been extremely traumatic and at times life-threatening, it also had had a sort of separate, dreamlike surrealism, whereas being home in New Zealand, which was going through a deep recession at the time, meant it was now time to front up and quit dwelling on my misery and start the long, slow trek up the mountain of my life and try to re-enter the everyday world.

28

Baby steps to recovery

Bear in mind that although it seemed like forever to me, I had only been totally drug-free for around eight months, so as far as taking actual pills was concerned, my nervous system was still not equipped, both biochemically or psychologically, to handle any stressful situation that had the potential to confuse or challenge me to any degree. The TRANX formula, that it could take my nervous system up to seven years to completely settle down from day one of the withdrawal process in Brisbane the previous year, meant that total recovery for me was still possibly at least six years away. But dwelling on my faulty, mental software wasn't going to serve any useful purpose if I was to get my life back on track, so it was onwards and upwards, regardless of how terrible I was feeling on any given day.

January 1993 arrived. It was now twelve months since I'd taken that initial plunge and started the process of going into withdrawal and self-detox in Brisbane and here I was, trapped alive, living with my mother, unemployed, ill and with no map of the future or what it was going to even look like. How much worse could it get? It's around this time in the scheme of things where you start to really believe in karma and think perhaps I must've done something horrible to a Chinaman in a previous life for mine to end up like this.

My instinct that living with my mother would motivate me to get going turned out to be correct.

Surviving on a few hours' sleep during the night and having her playing mind games with me by day came to a head within a short space of time, so I moved out to rent my own small bedsitter room in a boarding house full of unusual people. Again, surrealism came nibbling in, as the boarding house was in a very wealthy, upmarket part of town with a spectacular view of the bay. By night, the ships and ocean liners would come and go from the Napier city port below, with their twinkling, fairy deck lights and the sounds of music and happy passengers drifting across the ether, whilst elsewhere, peering through an invisible veil of wistfulness like a sad squirrel, there was me, living a very distinctly down-market existence gazing out from my forlorn little window high up on the hill above the port.

I was starting to run low on what little money I had left, so the time came for me to apply for government assistance just to get by and keep the wolf from the door. Because of my circumstances, I qualified for a sickness benefit, which paid slightly more than the standard benefit, but to get it I needed to have a doctor's certificate, so I went back to the local doctor who, funnily enough, was the second medical professional to prescribe me benzos 13 years earlier.

He was very sympathetic and apologetic and some months later when I instituted proceedings of medical misadventure under the government Accident Compensation Corporation (ACC) system, he was one of the few who gave documented evidence that I had, indeed, suffered misadventure (but more about that later).

Applying for a welfare benefit is a very demeaning thing to undergo and it only serves to make you feel more useless and lower than you already do. I found myself filling in a lengthy questionnaire before being interviewed by a fat, balding benefit officer who appeared to have the attention span of a sheep. Halfway through his insulting and probing questions, I started to spin out and go into a state of panic, so he must've been quite puzzled when I suddenly stood up and walked out without saying a word.

This didn't seem to faze the system because I made an appointment a few days later and they rubber-stamped my sickness benefit application. It was only about NZ$200 weekly and most of it was going on rent, but at least it slowed down the steady bleeding of what money I had left. I learnt long ago that the trick when you're under great pressure is to not focus on the macro picture of your situation, as it will just swamp you and take you down further below the baseline. No, the trick is to compartmentalise the immediate problems needing to be addressed for survival and work your way through them one at a time, consequently keeping the pressure down, which is how I managed my finances. How weird my life had become!

So, there I was. Needing a job, holed up in a small garret and trying to figure out my next moves. Finding a job was going to be the hardest challenge but I did have an ace up my sleeve, which I guarded like a precious jewel.

As you will recall earlier in my story, I had lived for a few years back in the same region that I had now returned to and in that previous time I had built up a good reputation in the retail advertising scene as a man who was media and marketing savvy. I'd had a stable of successful businessmen from back then who respected my ability to put things together and to make them money.

I was living a long way under the radar since returning this time and no one of any consequence knew I was back, but I understood that if I could ever get myself into a situation where I could call on those whom I'd dealt with in the past, then that would give me a head start.

Consequently, it was important that I didn't squander my past reputation by just taking any job, such as selling advertising on drink coasters or door-to-door encyclopaedias, as those bottom-dweller types of work were always available for the desperate.

Even though it meant I was living very frugally, I stayed staunch until I was offered a job selling Motorola cellphones. Bear in mind that this was the nineties, and the days of *Miami Vice*-type phones the size of bricks were very fashionable and it was all new technology, but I gave it a go on a small retainer plus commission. I didn't have an office or any such luxury; just a desk beside the lavatory out the back of the company premises.

I managed to generate sales but the anxiety levels of cold calling and trying to explain the intricacies of new technology (which I hardly understood myself) to tradesmen and doctors soon spun me out, so after a couple of tense, anxious months I had to fold up my tent and pack it in. Still, baby steps in the right direction as the wheels of my life gradually turned forward and my neural pathways were fed a slow diet of new thinking in an equally new Ativan-free state of mind.

Not long after leaving the cellphone job, I got a phone call from a local businessman whom I'd pitched a mobile phone proposition to. He asked me if I'd be interested in joining a new business publication being produced by one of the major local newspapers. It was a salaried sales position with a decent office and was located near to where I was living in my garret. Feigning indifference, I told him I'd think about it but I was, of course, delighted by this new development and I took it, as it was pulling me, respectably, back into the arena of advertising and marketing where I had previously enjoyed some level of kudos.

Things went well for a while but again I found my cognitive processes were still not up to speed or serving me correctly. There was a female staff member in the office where there was mutual dislike and I found everything too much, too soon, so again after a few months of doing a good job creating sales, I had to call it a day. Unfortunately, under New Zealand employment law if you willingly resign from your job for no acceptable reasons, you have a six-month stand-down period before you can again get government assistance, unless suffering from some type of disability, so I was left with no choice but to troop back to the sympathetic doctor and go back on the soul-destroying welfare sickness benefit.

Casting my mind back to the 12 steps of NA (and AA), I now realise why one of the earlier steps was that 'you are not to form any relationships with members of the opposite sex or emotional bonds for two years' — yep, two years. The reasoning behind this step, as I said earlier in the book, was that the initial joy and blush of meeting a new girlfriend or re-entering society before you were emotionally and psychologically ready and had at least two years' drug-free experience under your belt, could cause you to over-invest your sense of self-confidence or sexual and emotional feelings into a situation that stood a good chance of failing, due to your state of mind. The big danger when things went sour was that it could reactivate all the old past hurts and open the 'hole in your soul' again that had led you to use drugs or alcohol in the first instance as a way of getting by. In other words, you stood the risk of hurtling back to where you were before you ever started in withdrawal and recovery and to start drinking or drugging again to offset the pain of failing at the first hurdle in the outside world.

In my case, I could've been forgiven for following that path of 'picking up' or relapsing again due to the crushing disappointment at failing to handle my two recent jobs, but because I'd always seen my previous time at Narcotics Anonymous as simply my way of embracing an infrastructure to wrap around me while I weaned myself off a chemical dependence, rather than my being a lost-boy addict, I wasn't tempted to start taking pills again.

Whilst the 12-steps programme in NA is a fantastic psychological blueprint for recovery from not only drugs but also a completely ruined life, I didn't see the steps (other than maybe the first four) as being relative to my overall journey. (I can hear some NA members reading this and going 'you're still in denial and not in recovery — just fooling yourself — get to a meeting'.)

But, no, I felt no compulsion to go back and drown my sorrows in a chemical, Ativan blanket. Far from it, as I knew full well that to go back was to die in all ways. However, I had by now been away long enough from the strict guidelines of NA to not be quite so averse to the occasional cold beer on a lonely night, so I licked my wounds from leaving my job by sucking on cheap beer as I gazed out the window from my bolthole, at the ships in the harbour and continued my journey upwards towards the light.

29

Transcendental meditation

Because I had time on my hands, I decided to spend some of my precious dollars on a gym membership. Exercise is one of the best ways to 'heal' the recovering brain structure, as it forces your brain, under exertion, to produce nature's cocaine, otherwise known as endorphins. So twice daily, morning and late afternoon, I could be found prancing around the local gym, which was a totally new concept to me. In a short space of time, I started to become fit, which ain't no bad thing. The main upside, other than the exercise, was that I also started making friends with various other characters at the gym, some of whom turned out to be in the same boat as me, which was fine as there was no sense of social hierarchal challenge.

The next big breakthrough in my odyssey was to spot an advertisement in the local newspaper inviting people to a free transcendental meditation seminar. For those of you who don't know what transcendental meditation (TM) is, you must have been living under a rock for most of your life.

This form of meditating was the one espoused by the Maharishi Yogi who catapulted to fame when The Beatles, especially George Harrison, discovered it in their acid-driven days and all duly trooped off to Rishikesh in India to sit at the feet of the Maharishi and learn this style of meditating.

It became very fashionable back then in the seventies and many other stars, such as some of The Beach Boys, Donovan and Mia Farrow, plus other celebrities joined the fun days of dope, songwriting and learning the ancient arts of India. All was peace, love and flowers until John Lennon found out that the naughty old Maharishi had been trying to touch up Mia Farrow who was, apparently, tantalisingly naked under her flowing kaftan. In disgust, Lennon wrote the famous song 'Sexy Sadie', which was a thinly veiled tilt at the guru, and they all packed up and left, except George Harrison who remained true to Eastern mysticism until his death many years later from lung cancer.

Following my instincts, I booked a seat at the seminar and was impressed by what it offered. It's all very trendy nowadays to focus on mindfulness and 'being in the moment', but essentially that's what meditating was going to train me to do. Calming down the 'monkey mind' swinging from branch to branch in my inner thoughts and clearing my mind of my past horror movie (otherwise known as my life in recovery) and the years before seemed to be a perfect concept. This was just the antidote I needed, so I signed up.

The downside was that it cost NZ$800 to take the full two-day weekend course to be held the following week.

That much money represented quite a chunk of what cash I had left from a small inheritance that I'd received from my father, but my instincts told me it was offering me another step on my path towards regaining some modicum of my former life, so I transcended the financial aspect in favour of enlightenment (sic). English author Somerset Maugham wrote a book called *The Razor's Edge* with the epigraph 'The path to salvation is as difficult to walk as the razor's edge' (paraphrased). This maxim resonated with me as certain synchronistic events started popping up in my world and transcendental meditation seemed to me to be one such touchstone that held the promise of taking me off that bloody razor's edge!

Signing up to TM turned out be a very smart move, as practising that style of meditation has served me extremely well right through my recovery and up to this very day. The process of learning at the two-day course was simple in its complexity. The teacher, a chirpy little bald man called Ian, basically explained the ancient Vedic knowledge behind the meditative process and then on the second day there was a charming induction process whereby you brought along a small offering of fruit and were 'blessed' and given your own personal mantra to use for focusing your mind when meditating, and that was basically it.

There's always been a global joke about the personal mantra, as you were solemnly told that under no circumstances were you ever to reveal it to anyone. The joke was that supposedly everyone, globally, had the exact same 'secret' personal mantra, but I never tested that out so I really don't know and didn't care, as the ritualistic side of the learning appealed to my sense of self.

The ongoing discipline was that you were to meditate twice daily every morning and evening, preferably before eating and strictly for only 20 minutes at a time. Each morning would find me, unemployed and nearly broke, sitting in my little room above the port trying to calm my mind and rotating the mantra in my head. Meditation (or mindfulness) is quite a challenge when you first get into it and, of course, doubly hard when your mind is in chaos, as mine had been for what seemed like an eternity. The trick was to not try to do or think anything. Just to simply let go of your thoughts whilst concentrating on your breathing and to focus only on the present moment, the *now* and what was happening inside and around you at that moment. When you think about it, it is *now* forever. It's not possible to be anything else! The past has vanished a second ago and the future is in the next second so it's always 'right now'. (*The Power of Now* by Eckhart Tolle is probably the best book on the subject.)

If you're doing your meditation correctly, the early days can be quite hard going as a lot of the troubled stuff from your past bubbles up from your subconscious, challenging you to address and reconcile the 'stuff', but because I'd already been confronted with most of those hellish demons in my stage two withdrawal period back in Australia, it wasn't too bad for me.

My days became quite pleasant whilst doing my TM discipline and even The Dark Shadow, which was always there, lurking around like a troglodyte within my deeper self, now seemed to have settled down to a dull roar, which gave me hope that I may be finally on the mend.

For some strange reason (probably searching out non-judgmental company), I had also occasionally taken to dropping into the local Anglican Church Cathedral and partaken in holy communion with an assortment of little old ladies and sanctimonious, lemon-lipped types. Mixed with the daily gym workout and my meditation, I started to feel a gradual sense of slowing of that spin cycle that my life had been on for what had seemed like forever.

But life was not about to stay peaceful for very long in my existence of brain defragging and dumping of my temporary mental files in the land of 'Om mani padme hum'. Because we often live our lives retrospectively, what may appear to be an absolutely disastrous situation can often turn out, in hindsight, to be a major breakthrough of the positive kind, which is exactly how things played out for me in the coming weeks.

The landlord of the boarding house where I lived at that time was some sort of sexually obsessed fruitcake who spent most of his days furtively peering out the window at school-girls passing by and apparently masturbating, as it turned out. He lived next to my upstairs bedsit and initially was quite pleasant and friendly, but for some strange, paranoid reason he suddenly took it upon himself to believe that all the tenants were sneaking into his rooms and stealing his money and his books. He began leaving cryptic notes under our doors, so the upshot of this madness was that very quickly the tenants, who weren't guilty of anything, started leaving.

I was unemployed, winter had arrived and I had nowhere to go. The stress of having this clown leaving me strange notes and prowling around my flat at night whilst I slept (he had keys) soon put me back into an understandable state of extremely high anxiety. The meditation, the gym and all the coping tools I'd learned in recovery flew out the window as I tried to handle this very threatening situation of being trapped without alternatives and the only small sense of security I had being threatened and eroded. His harassment rapidly came to a head. It got to the point of my recognising the anxiety-overload danger signals within myself and my very being starting to fall to pieces with the likelihood of all my good work over the past 18 months virtually going out the door!

In desperation, I had rung my friend Margie back in Mullumbimby, Australia, to tell her that I'd tried my best in the outside world but I just couldn't handle it with all its daily challenges whilst still trying to completely recover, and that after the pressure I'd been through, my only viable option was to go back to Australia and face the fact that my old life, as I knew it, as a successful human being, was gone and that the time had come for me to pay the price for my 13 years of accidental Ativan addiction and everything that came before that in my previous life. But then a very strange thing happened!

As I was starting the slow grind of getting it together and dejectedly preparing to leave the country, the phone rang. It was an ex-girlfriend ringing to say 'hi' but when she quickly ascertained that I was not in a good space and was staring down the barrel of nowhere to live, she said the words that were to begin the change in direction that would end up leading me from the very bottom of the heap to eventually becoming a millionaire and living a life that I could never have imagined.

Yes, dear readers — we have now turned the corner of my continuous story of negativity and misery. The good news and the reward for going to hell and back to break my addiction was soon going to manifest itself in my changing world, and the unfolding story from here on will, hopefully, give you the inspiration to start for yourself the long, arduous process of benzo withdrawal and eventual happy recovery in a life you could only guess at back in those miserable, addicted days.

PART III

Into the Light

30

Case studies of benzo sadness

Some of the survivors of benzo dependency have been successful in not only overcoming their addiction but also receiving monetary compensation. A gentleman named Ray Nimmo, who lived in Great Britain, started the excellent benzobuddies.org website. His story began in 1984 when, after having an allergic reaction to an antibiotic, he was told by his doctor that the abdominal pain he was experiencing was just a muscle spasm and he was prescribed Xanax (a benzo) as a muscle relaxant. When Xanax failed to address the problem, Valium was prescribed and his downward spiral into addiction began for the next 14 years. As Ray put it himself during an interview on the BBC in 2002, 'I was suicidally depressed, so anxious, agoraphobic, lethargic. I just didn't want to go out of the house. I didn't want to answer the door or the telephone. I was just like a zombie.'

Unable to work, Ray lived in a 'twilight world of paranoia

and fear'. His doctors then told him that he was suffering from a mental illness and he trusted that prognosis, as doctors knew best (where have I heard that before?).

It was only in 1998 that another doctor, a surgeon at a local hospital, examining Ray after an ultrasound treatment, told him that his problems were due to being on Valium (diazepam). Another doctor confirmed this view and diagnosed him as having Valium-induced depression as well as a chronic Valium addiction. With this doctor's guidance, Ray gradually reduced his intake of drugs over the next three months. The agoraphobia, anxiety and suicidal depression he had suffered for over 14 years were eventually resolved. Feeling like his old self again and determined to get redress for the injustice of having had 14 years of his life ruined, Ray Nimmo sued the physician who had kept him on drugs for all that time. He was awarded £40,000 in 2002 and went on to become a champion for the cause of benzodiazepine over-prescription in the United Kingdom.

He also developed and curated the *benzo.org.uk* website, and initiated the BenzoBuddies Community Forum (http://www.benzobuddies.org/forum/) online community where fellow victims of benzodiazepine dependence could go to share their experiences of withdrawal and, hopefully, eventual recovery. However, I should warn you it is not pretty reading in a lot of instances and should be approached with caution. The reason for this is that, although well intentioned and true, some of the live postings on this forum are so heartbreaking that they could put you off taking the initial steps needed to free yourself from the curse of addiction. Also, these sorts of forums can become addictive within themselves and, under the auspices of 'misery loves company', you can end up with counterproductive advice and stay trapped down there on misery street. However, it's up to you, as there are also many stories of people making it to freedom available in the forums and some great information on this excellent and comprehensive site.

Here is a real-life, real-time excerpt from the BenzoBuddies forum written by a woman on 5 October 2016, who was taking Ativan and freaking out:

I am a new member of this forum as of today. And I am scared! I will be as brief as possible —

In July this past year after some health issues with my back and personal issues, complete with muscle twitches in legs, head, and arms, I had sort of what I categorize as a breakdown of sorts.

My then physician tried me on Zoloft, and I reacted badly. Then because I wasn't sleeping at all, trazadone, which was the same, bad. I was placed on generic Ativan, at 0.5 to 1mg a day as needed for anxiety. I take it only as prescribed. I never thought of a possibility of dependency until a few days ago.

I had noticed that about mid-afternoon if I took a dose in the night before that I would get uptight and crying, almost on a daily basis. A few weeks ago, I didn't take it for a few days and my anxiety jumped through the roof, my twitches went through the roof, and my arms and legs would 'jump'. My body on two occasions felt locked up. I went to my doctor who after all the tests I have went through also did an MRI of my brain. Nothing.

Fast forward to now. I haven't taken any Ativan since the morning before yesterday. Yesterday the twitches and anxiety returned, almost to a panic. I am so scared — I never have drunk alcohol or used any drugs before.

What if I have developed a dependence? Does this sound like it to anyone, even though I only used it as prescribed, since this past early July — about 5 days a week on average? The muscle twitches, jerks, headaches, stomach aches, increased anxiety withdrawal??

Like I said, at 39 years old, I have never drunk alcohol, used drugs, or misused medications and I am scared! I so want to be a good wife and mom, and certainly don't want to be a slave to this type of fear. I want my life back!!! Thank you, and blessings!

Tragically for her, this woman has not been given any medical advice by her prescribing doctor as to what she is doing, which is putting her in a dangerous state of constant withdrawal from the Ativan due to the fact that she is not following a consistent, daily dose and consequently is on a nightmare roller-coaster ride.

This illustrates nothing's changed over the last 55 years since benzos first hit the market. I can fully understand what this woman is posting above, having had similar experiences when I was in withdrawal and self-detox, and it angers me to see that some of the medical profession don't get it and are still making potential addicts out of innocent people.

31

The arrival of the cavalry

We've now, hopefully, established that what I have written about up to this point in my book about benzo/tranquilliser addiction is not just exclusive to me but a story shared by millions of everyday people around the world, one way or another. But now the nasty stuff is thankfully behind me in my unfolding tale.

It's funny how your life can turn on a dime from achingly hopeless to vaguely hopeful. After more than two years in the abyss of addiction and recovery fallout, my friendly card seemed to have finally arrived.

As you will recall, in a previous chapter I was right up against the wall and preparing to just give in, 'fold up my tent', head back to Australia and oblivion and now, with just one phone call from a woman friend, my circumstances were about to change irrevocably.

When I told her that I would shortly have nowhere to live,

she asked me if I knew a well-known local Chinese businessman, Harry Deng, who owned a palatial property at the top of the best street in the most expensive real estate in the region. I most certainly did and had done good business for him when I previously lived in the Bay, handling the radio advertising for his chain of women's fashion outlets. Apparently, Harry had a small but luxurious, fully furnished, poolside cabana at the back of his property and it was becoming vacant. My ex-girlfriend suggested I gave Harry a call and see whether I could meet up with him, which I promptly did. He definitely remembered me and our business connections so he was happy for me to come over to his mansion and check out the property.

If I'd had wings I would've flown there immediately but trying to sound laid-back about it all, I made a time and duly turned up the next day and there it was in all its resplendent glory (or that's how it looked to me after my proverbial '40 days in the wilderness' of life).

Surrounded by beautiful gardens, looking out over green lawns and a large, crystal-clear swimming pool, was my next abode and the first step into a yet-to-be-discovered, brilliant future. Harry casually said that if I liked it, it was mine for NZ$120 a week, including power. Unbelievable!

From the stance of the anxiety–ridden world I'd occupied for the last two years, this place looked like a cross between a hospital pass and paradise, so I shook his hand and the deal was done. I got back to the dump I was living in and left a note for the crazy landlord, giving notice that I was leaving his madhouse. He slipped a note back under my door in response, riddled with abuse and a line that I've always smiled about when my life eventually improved beyond belief.

It said, 'You'll be lucky to find anywhere from here onwards where you won't be staring out a small window at a tin fence in some miserable dump!' Yes, he was a charmer and I often wonder what became of him, but, quite frankly, I don't give a damn!

And, no, I never ever did meet up with that tin fence. In fact, I eventually ended up owning a three-storey mansion with an elevator, views to the mountains surrounded by lush green trees at the top of a private driveway. But we'll get to that later.

Since that phone call that changed my life and 'para-chuted' me into my own personal oasis of peace and calm, it would be easy to think that the magic wand had been waved and all my ongoing inner turmoil and daily anxiety had been resolved. No such luck. Having somewhere secure and peaceful to live was a major breakthrough in providing me with the first signs in the last two to three years of any semblance of balance and sanity returning to my life, but 'one swallow does not a summer make', as the saying goes. In other words, I was still unemployed, on a sickness benefit and running on a flawed but gradually recovering circuitry in my brain. I guess the main thing I had to contend with was the constant ongoing, relentless and unnecessary over-blown anxiety.

However, having finally found a break in the traffic and been washed up onto a haven of serenity and peace in the shape of my new-found abode, I felt a sense of safety for the first time in many, many moons, which helped towards the calming of the brain processes and to the general improvement of my state of mind.

With help from a friend, I moved what little I had into the cabana. To sit in my comfortable lounge looking out at a sparkling, clear swimming pool, framed by manicured gardens, was something like a dream wish from Aladdin's lamp. Spring had arrived and I can remember buying a simple bunch of newly-burst daffodils and putting them in a slender, white vase that I'd had stored and then placing them on a glass-topped coffee table in the lounge. It may seem odd to some people, but as I sat in the silence of the approaching dusk of evening, looking at the sheer, beautiful simplicity of a freshly cut bunch of flowers, I quietly wept. Not in pain but in relief and gratitude that after being in a maelstrom of insanity for so long surrounded by addicts, madness and potential death that at last I stood a faint chance of resurrecting some semblance of a liveable life.

That life continued to roll along as life inevitably does and nothing stays the same for ever. I was starting to feel better in that I'd now been drug-free long enough for my cerebral cortex and hippocampus to start the marvel of neuro-plasticity and begin to lay down fresh, untainted neural pathways based on the new concepts being presented by my daily existence.

The neural pathways in the brain are a very important factor in getting your thinking back on track. The brain is structured so that when you have a thought that is negative and depressing and you keep rethinking it, like the donkey going round and around the well until it wears down a familiar groove, your brain starts laying down a 'thought highway' so the more you think about negative things or your ex-girlfriend or whatever; the more that highway gets embedded in your mind until it starts automatically delivering into your consciousness what it thinks you want. You wake up in the morning, the negative thought pattern drops into the slot like a pinball machine and soon you've defined your upcoming day as a total downer. By making a real effort to delete any such negative thoughts as soon as they enter your mind you can re-program your thought patterns so that eventually those deep, negative neural pathways will start to revert backwards until they become 'bush tracks' and then they're gone. You can control your thinking and that's how it works. And, of course, it works in reverse with positive thoughts.

Largely because sleeplessness and nightmares were still a big issue for me and with my faith in the medical profession all but gone, I started to sniff around the alternative medicine scene for answers to my circumstances. I consulted a very sincere old homeopath lady, and for a while I was taking everything from nux vomica for my personality, aurum metallicum for my apparently broken heart, arsenicum to flush the poisons from my system, kali phos for the nerves, and much more. Those of you that know homeopathy will understand when I say that I really don't know what worked or if in fact it even did, but it was all part of my gradual daily grind to keep occupied and crawl slowly upwards to the light, and was surely worth a shot. I would recommend Bach Flowers Rescue Remedy when you're in the early stages of withdrawal.

Each day, I'd hit the gym and in the afternoons, I'd climb high in the volcanic hills behind where I lived. Not only did this help exhaust me, which assisted in getting much-needed nightly sleep, but the famous Wordsworth poetry line of 'I wandered lonely as a cloud' had the sublime effect of nourishing my inner soul, plus there was always a chance of fulfilling his poem *Daffodils* by finding some fresh ones growing wild in the country!

During my earlier attempt at working for the business magazine when I first arrived back in the Bay, I had been hooked up with a heavily subsidised employee health insurance scheme which I had kept paying into. This gave me access to psychologists, entitling me to a claimable rebate of most of the cost, so I decided it was time to continue the final purging of the leftover fragments of addiction withdrawal recovery, stage two. As I explained earlier, I originally thought that the initial detox of the drug in my system would be a compressed, intense trip to hell and back but that would be the end of it. Actually, I hate to say it but the physical horrors of initial withdrawal are in some ways the easy bit. You're vomiting, trembling, hallucinating and generally flying to pieces, but you know what's happening to you and why.

I found a local shrink and in we went again, to the inner world of Rob Pharazyn and the disassembled, cognitive labelling of my emotions.

32

Tangling with bureaucracy

Those who have undergone therapy will know what I mean when I say that my new-found chum, the shrink, was your stereotypical psychologist. Bearded, dressed in clashing-coloured clothes and possessed of a tone of voice that was a cross between talking to a dog that had just been run over and a human being (me) who was less than perfect but needed soothing, by sounding like you were offering him (me) some calming type of soup.

It's a clever thing is your psychological counselling, because essentially all they do is get you to rave on about your hidden fears and anxieties from childhood onwards whilst they sit there saying very little and jotting something down on a notepad while the money-meter silently clicks on by till your hour is up. Any time you ask them a question, they invariably ask you the same question prefaced by 'What do you think?', which means you must keep unloading. But it works. Knowing that you're talking under the guarantee of confidentiality allows you to dive deep into the darker recesses of your psyche and the mere process of verbalising those fears and horrors seems to defragment the brain and create space for new and up-to-date thinking, which is what I needed.

I visited him once a week for about nine months, but having spent a lot of time with Dr Zed, my main man shrink a few years back in Australia who had nearly incinerated my mind in the end, I felt I'd already covered a lot of the deep stuff, so this new head-doctor was really nothing much more than a sounding board to reassure me that I was on the right track and that I was not just an ungrateful lout who harboured uncharitable thoughts about his mother! There was only so long I could listen to him while sitting in his rooms, pondering his Roman sandals and his constant stroking of his beard, so eventually I stopped going and that was the last time I took on therapy of any sort — ever!

My everyday life had become a less than exciting rotate of walks, gym, reading, eating, meditating and then bed for a storm-tossed kind of sleep and then 'get up in de mornin', 'same ting for breakfast' and away I would go for another soulless day. I would scour the job section in the local paper but nothing much of any promise appeared and, by now, I was getting desperate for my future way of ever earning any money to get me back into some semblance of a reasonable life.

In New Zealand, the government has a system that applies to all citizens, which covers you for almost anything that could go wrong with you, physically or mentally. It's called the Accident Compensation Corporation and in exchange for abdicating any rights to litigate for any problems you incur, the ACC would look after you in the form of a bulk payout or subsidised wages for an extended period if you were unable to work due to some injury or disabling misfortune.

Back then, under the category of 'medical misadventure', ACC had been paying out sizeable chunks of cash settlements to women (or men) who claimed to have been sexually abused but had repressed the terrible event to the point that they'd forgotten it had ever happened to them! Consequently, it became a growth industry to suddenly remember someone 'feeling you up', etc. when you were a kid and now, as an adult, walking off with an average payout of 10K without ever having to supply any evidence, except your version of what you'd suddenly and miraculously remembered. As you can imagine, this became a very popular pastime but it also scooped up some poor unfortunate and innocent individuals in its net who were falsely accused, just to get the payout through and into the pocket of the accuser.

However, under the same medical misadventure category I discovered that ACC had been paying out, albeit begrudgingly, up to 50K cash settlements to people who over the last 30 years had been prescribed benzodiazepine tranquillisers by doctors, without ever being advised of the addictive properties and the ongoing mental fallout from such an addiction when any attempts were made at stopping the medication. This described my situation to a tee.

Synchronicity kicked in and I discovered a man working locally who had received such a payout, so I made time to chat with him and find out how to go about seeing if I could get some form of money from ACC to help me survive until

I could get back to gainful employment and a steady income. He told me that, unfortunately, he was at the tail end of the payouts and that ACC were closing the gates unless you could provide irrefutable proof of being prescribed tranquillisers without any follow-up warnings, etc., but he was invaluable in taking me through the procedures required.

I contacted ACC who duly sent me out a mind-numbingly large pile of questionnaires and forms to wade my way through, but time was something I had plenty of, so I sat down for about two weeks and went right back to the first doctor's visit (described at the beginning of this book) and all the other doctors who had ever prescribed Ativan to me. As you can imagine, this was one hell of a task as I'd moved around a lot but, methodically, I worked my way from day one till when I started self-detoxification in Australia in the nineties and provided all the details. (Remember that I didn't have the luxury of Google or a laptop, which is hard to imagine, seeing it wasn't really that far back to the mid-nineties.)

Along with the huge amount of paperwork, I had to present a personal submission as to why ACC should consider my case for compensation and I think it is revealing for me to give you the final page of that lengthy submission:

There are many after-effects to my situation but the bottom line is that my life is slowly 'bleeding' away and although I make every endeavour to improve it, only the Gods can save me from a very mediocre existence at best.

Whilst my natural psychology played a part in my scenario, I consider my unsolicited exposure to the benzodiazepine drug, Ativan, to be responsible for my current, ongoing predicament and that no prescribing doctor, bar one, ever tried to warn me of the dangers or prevent my usage even though the addictive qualities and dangers were well-documented before my first prescription. Money is not really the issue here although some compensation would enable me to continue along my path of recovery with a better chance of success.

My logic in this lengthy submission is that I would not willingly throw away a rewarding radio career, the only woman I've loved, my sanity and my health plus a large amount of lost earnings in exchange for this pathetic, lonely existence as a recovering addict and a near penniless social alien!

At least the hardcore junkies got some thrills from their drug use and addiction but have you ever heard of closet benzo users throwing get together parties?

I realise that apparently not all benzo users suffer as I have but that doesn't really provide solace to me. I can produce witnesses and details to cover the whole sorry story of the past nearly 15 years which includes my detox and recovery period to date and can substantiate any details of the trauma I have suffered through no fault of my own.

I state categorically, that if I had been told by the first prescribing doctor about the known facts surrounding usage of Ativan I would not have taken them as I was only seeking a remedy for sleeplessness back then.

I now live every millisecond of my anxiety driven, sparse existence and it is not pleasant. The real me sits quietly beneath the storm of my daily life, waiting patiently as my physiology and psychology continues to betray me!

Even though I wrote that some years ago, I can still clearly remember the winter's afternoon, hunched over the kitchen table, putting the submission together in my own handwriting, with little or no idea of what was to come not very far down the line.

33

Medical misadventure?

The wheels of justice move slowly and so do government departments. It was about six weeks before I got a response, which was couched in babbling legalese and bureaucratic jargon, probably in an effort to deter me.

I decided the easy answer was to find a lawyer who could unpick things and represent me. I'd had a brief, past acquaintance with a leading lawyer from one of the top law firms, so I made time to go and see him to present my story. He was sympathetic and kindly offered to only send a bill after any outcomes and would view it based on a pro bono basis if I got financial compensation from ACC.

What a rigmarole! Over the next 12 months, paper flew backwards and forwards between the Corporation and my lawyer as we steadily batted away their attempts to blindside my application for a judgment based on my being a victim of medical misadventure.

Twice, they sent an investigator up from Wellington, the capital city of New Zealand and about four hours' drive away, to put me through the hoops on my details to try to trip me up and push me back from any chance of success.

The meetings with the investigator were like something you'd expect when being interrogated by the Russian KGB. They took place in a very large, empty room in a high-rise office block. In the middle of the room were a table and a wooden chair where I sat, with my protagonist opposite me taking notes whilst a small tape recorder whirred away. He was polite and friendly, but was not there to waste time on pleasantries.

In my original submission, I'd provided, to the best of my ability, the names of every doctor within New Zealand who had ever prescribed me benzos but, unfortunately, I couldn't remember the name of the doctor who had first prescribed the Ativan in my one, brief medical centre visit 16 years earlier. (ACC later seized on this point as a reason to not accept my claim.)

After a period, the ACC system started spewing out reams of paper to my lawyer, including letters of response from all the doctors that I had named in my submission. I still have these copies and they make for very interesting reading as doctor after doctor tried to dodge the bullet of responsibility. Amusingly, some tried to blame me for their lack of diligence when prescribing me with benzos. One said in his response to ACC:

'I find that his stated unawareness and lack of insight into the possible harmful side-effects of benzodiazepines as being a little inconsistent with his obvious degree of intelligence and experience as a top rating radio talkback host.'

Another doctor, in his submission response, said, amongst other comments:

'... that Mr. Pharazyn's impressive appearance and verbal fluency would make the task of refusing his requests for prescriptions, very difficult.'

Interestingly, the doctor who was the second one to ever prescribe me Ativan way back at the start, said in his submission response that:

'... it is my belief that the ongoing prescription of benzodiazepines to a person of Mr. Pharazyn's age [not sure what age has to do with it as I was only in my late twenties back then] knowing as we do now of their addictive properties, probably constitutes medical misadventure.'

It's hard to know what to say about that, as the whole issue underpinning this book is that overall, in my opinion, the medical profession is probably more culpable in the massive benzo addiction problem than the drug companies that supply the pills, and now here we have a doctor being honest enough to admit that prescribing benzos was an unwise thing to do to me.

Sure, Big Pharma and the drug companies are only interested in shareholder profits and will pump drugs onto the market that can make a buck, but without the doctors prescribing them there's no circular money-go-round and pipeline. This is why the drug companies woo doctors with all-expenses-paid trips to foreign countries, staying in five-star hotels, with the only reciprocal obligation on the doctor's part being to listen to a short presentation on drug X, collect their free Mont Blanc fountain pen and then go have fun. Next time you're at a doctor's surgery, have a look at the brand names on their desk pad, pens, etc. — all drug companies!

I'm not, by any means, suggesting that all physicians are incompetent or servants of the major drug companies. Far from it. I'm simply highlighting the way the big drug companies inveigle doctors into viewing their product more favourably. Surely doctors must believe in the drugs they use to treat us and surely, it's not too much to expect to trust that our doctors have our best interests covered, but I do question the lack of treating the actual person, not just the complaint and the casual handing out of prescriptions for drugs. I think it's reasonable for us to expect doctors to have thoroughly checked out the benefits and side effects of a drug before prescribing it, and not just unquestioningly prescribe drugs that have been clearly shown to have harmful side effects or highly addictive properties. It's that '*Primum non nocere* — first do no harm' thing again, which is the oath that doctors take.

Without boring you with all the details of the ping-pong paper shuffle over months between ACC and my lawyer, I'll now move on to their final attempt to unravel me.

ACC had considered all the responses from the doctors and my replies and, to date, had rejected my claim three times. But we kept on coming at them. They now took the gloves off and went to Plan B, which was to commission an independent report from a psychiatrist at the Hastings DHB Hospital Psychiatric Unit NZ (you'd think I'd have had enough by now but morbid fascination drove me on).

As directed, at 9am on Saturday, 18 March 1995 I turned up at the office of a shrink called Tim Florrit for my next interrogation (not therapy, I hasten to add). According to the notes I received later, his brief was to report on (to quote ACC):

1. What symptoms and difficulties have arisen from the bodily effects of Mr. Pharazyn's withdrawal from Ativan?

2. In the period between his first exposure to Ativan and prior to his ceasing taking the drug, which of the difficulties and symptoms Mr. Pharazyn experienced were due to taking Ativan, as opposed to any underlying conditions and influences, in both the present and the past, in Mr. Pharazyn's life? (like, was Mr. Pharazyn plain nuts anyway?)

3. Of those symptoms and difficulties which Mr. Pharazyn experienced and which he attributes to Ativan; would these symptoms or adverse consequences occur in more than 1% of cases where Ativan is prescribed?

Tim Florrit was not a bad chap and showed kindness and consideration towards me. His answers to the ACC's guidelines were very telling and you would've thought they'd have been most beneficial to my claim but, no, to the contrary.

Here are his findings relating to the ACC question mandate:

Q1: It is difficult to be specific about the symptoms and difficulties having arisen from the bodily effects of withdrawal from Ativan that Mr. Pharazyn experienced, as there were so many.

Q2: It is my opinion (Dr Florrit) that during the period Mr. Pharazyn was taking benzodiazepines (Ativan), most of his problems were, in fact, related to benzodiazepine addiction and not any of his previous life experiences!

Q3: It is my opinion (Dr Florrit) that the symptoms and difficulties arising from Mr. Pharazyn's Ativan addiction, would occur in more than 1% of cases where Ativan was prescribed.

ACC were probably not too happy that their tame shrink

hadn't played ball, but like the cunning little ferrets that they were, they found an out clause which was just pure bureau-crat-speak!

Their response was that the Review Committee, on the evidence before them:

'... *finds that the symptoms and adverse consequences experienced by Mr. Pharazyn would occur in more than 1% of cases where the drug was prescribed. This therefore would not satisfy the rarity criteria laid down in the medical misadventure act.*

'The committee accepts Mr. Pharazyn was severely disabled by the events which happened to him from benzodiazepines but this does not satisfy the rarity criteria of the Act and there is no evidence to establish medical error. Our committee recommendation is that his claim should be declined to become final within 15 working days.'

You couldn't make this stuff up!

So, because more than 1% of people who had been prescribed benzos (or Ativan, as I had been) suffered the horrors that I went through, it meant that it *wasn't* rare enough, which consequently made it somehow okay? I still shake my head at that logic and can't find any skerrick of reason in that the rarity context was the basis for declining my compensation claim for being prescribed a drug for 13 years without ever being given a warning of what continuous use could do in the form of addiction.

However, this declining of my application was just stage two of the game and the beginning of the standard ACC 'cat and mouse' modus operandi.

In other cases where applicants had been successful in getting compensated for claims to ACC for 'having suffered personal injury by accident through medical misadventure due to lack of appropriate warning by a doctor concerning the possibility of benzodiazepine addiction and the adverse effects flowing from that and that even if they were, the extent of the warning was insufficient' (the official definition) they had all been rejected until a third appeal, then those who were tenacious enough to get that far were rewarded as the money-tree usually gave forth and you were paid your rightful compensation.

The payouts were generally 50K for those that had ploughed on undaunted and filed appeals to the higher body of the Accident Compensation Appeal authority which, in my case, would've meant that the original findings and declining of my personal submission would most likely have been overturned on appeal and I may have been financially compensated, even though they'd supposedly closed the gates on payouts a while back. But it wasn't to be.

34

Back to work

In the real world, the continuous unfolding of my life had started to slowly swing towards the positive in its journey from hell to eventual happiness, but it would still take a bit more time to manifest itself to what it would eventually become; namely, a good life.

Over the slow grind of the many months that it took to wash through the government system, my ACC submissions were now just a background adjunct to my everyday life of living in my poolside cabana, doing my usual daily routine whilst still trying to get some form of employment and my life back on track.

Then my lawyer who was handling my ACC claim dropped a bombshell.

He phoned me and asked me to come into his office, as he needed to discuss things with me, which of course excited me, thinking that some major breakthrough in my case had arrived.

However, when I sat down with him he informed me that, firstly, he'd sought advice and, in all likelihood, I would win my claim for compensation on appeal, but for personal reasons he couldn't proceed to handle my case because, as it turned out, he was a very good friend of that bastard Dr Dan of yesteryear who had overdosed me with drugs and nearly incinerated my brain back in the late eighties (not to be confused with the Gold Coast shrink, Dr Zed, who, five years later, had also nearly fried my mind with chemicals — sigh).

My lawyer said if he proceeded he would have to put Dr Dan on the witness stand and rip him to shreds, as his actions were quite pivotal to winning my ACC claim and he said he just couldn't do it to a close friend and recommended a competent fellow lawyer from another firm who could take up my case and proceed. I don't know whether what he did to me was ethical, at the very least, or allowable by the Law Society, but that was just the latest twist and turn in my unusual life at that time.

I was completely blown away by this change of events. I went home and watched the sun go down over a cold beer and thought, 'Stuff it, I've had enough. This is the gods telling me to walk away, give it up, Rob, move on' and at that point my attempts to get what was probably due to me in financial compensation were finished. I'd had enough of going backwards and forwards reliving those horrible days in that chapter of my life. Angels apparently never know it's time to close the book and gracefully decline, but this tired angel knew it was now time to pull the pin. It was over!

One day, not long after that, I saw an advertisement in the

local, regional daily newspaper that was to lead me to where I am today: wealthy, drug and debt-free and in total control of all aspects of my life. Yes, the miracle resurrection of Mr Rob was about to commence. The warm jets were ready to be turned on and the gods had arrived!

The job advert read:

'Wanted. An experienced person to successfully edit, sell advertising, maintain the administration and clean the offices of a local fortnightly newspaper. A salary of 20K is offered, subject to review based on performance after two weeks.'

Two weeks, I thought wryly. That wasn't giving me much time to turn the ship around.

Nobody in their right mind would normally apply for a position which appeared to want the near impossible, but I wasn't really in my right mind after the last couple of years of high-stakes weirdness and was also in the unusual position of having absolutely nothing to lose by applying, as my current existence was going nowhere. So, I sent in an application with my CV and references. Given that my work history was one of being a high achiever in media and marketing, Abe, the newspaper's owner, must've fallen off his seat with excitement when he received my application, little knowing what my life had actually been like recently.

He invited me in for an interview, so I put on a suit and tie like the good old days, slipping my gold Longines watch on my wrist, looking every inch a successful applicant, and off I went to meet Abe. He was a small man dressed in old clothes, beads of anxiety-driven sweat on his brow and baled up in a small upstairs office that was co-shared by a stern-looking woman who seemed to be offering services in laminating documents (and probably spankings, judging by her looks).

It definitely wasn't what I'd expected. Although I had no knowledge of the publishing or printing industry, this didn't seem to me to be much more than a hobby paper.

I'd done some background due diligence on the business and knew that the paper owed money to the tax department, plus other angry local creditors. It seemed that it was staggering along on its last legs and was pretty much on the verge of closing. I asked him how he proposed to pay me and that's when he told me that he'd finance my salary out of his 'bumblebee money'. His what?

Abe, who not only endeavoured to publish the paper each fortnight, also appeared to try to pay the bills by catching bumblebees (you may need to Google that, depending on which country you're in) at the weekends.

His method was to go roaming with his butterfly net to nearby rivers and selected places around the local countryside where certain types of bush, mainly lupins, were in flower. He'd have a small detachable plastic capsule attached on the end of the net and as he caught a bee off a flower, he'd transfer them to a bigger container until he had collected a sizeable amount.

He'd then store the container full of agitated bumblebees in his refrigerator at home. The bees would go into a slumber and when the daily price of bees went up to a profitable level he'd take them out, feed them some honey-water to reactivate them and onsell them to a big operator. Sort of like a stock exchange, but for bees! You may ask what was the point in all this bee-napping? It turns out that there is good money selling bumblebees to nurseries etc. for pollination purposes so Abe made a buck and the bumblebees went to a bee heaven of blooming flowers.

As you can imagine, I felt like it was back down the rabbit hole time, all over again, upon being informed that technically I was going to be paid in bumblebees if I took the job, but I'd been down so many blind alleys of late that my curiosity got the better of me and I pressed on for more details. I asked him about the debt ratio of the business and quite how he expected me to do virtually everything involved in running the paper and make it successful in just two weeks? He waved that aside and said if I wanted the job, it was mine, and could I start yesterday? The whole scenario was so bizarre that it appealed to my sense of the absurd and fitted into my current life's erratic tapestry. One major plus was that the business was on life support and near collapse, so there was only one way forward and that was up. No matter what I did, there was no great expectation or pressure on me to be an immediate boy wonder. I accepted the job to start the following Monday.

It was June and the New Zealand winter had appeared with a vengeance. Early Monday morning duly arrived with my alarm clock jangling me awake to the sound of a rainstorm howling around outside. At that moment, I thought, 'This is a waste of time working for a nearly dead newspaper. I think I'll go back to sleep under these nice, warm blankets', but the phone rang and it was a friend calling to wish me luck on my first day.

I often smile at how close I came to never having a rendezvous with my successful destiny. If that friend hadn't rung and I'd just gone back to sleep and not turned up for my first day at the office, it's hard to know what my future would've become.

The newspaper office was open plan and not furnished with anything much more than the basics. My desk was nearly falling over but it had a working phone and there was a fax machine, so at least the basic tools were there for me to start marketing to the outside world. There were two computers, with one being used to compose very basic versions of the few advertisements that were still coming in and the other one was for a freelance writer who was being paid a pittance for each supplied story. The actual production of the paper was so primitive that everything editorially was converted from the computer to the copy machine and then cut and pasted into hard copy. Next step was to cut and paste the editorial body copy of the paper with a glue stick and a Stanley knife onto pre-formatted sheets, which were eventually scanned and converted to film and then printed by the local printers. Hard to believe that this was only 20 years ago, but I had no knowledge of printing so I saw it as an opportunity to learn from the ground up. It was really bizarre but at the same time hugely amusing.

35

Becoming Rupert Murdoch?

My work rhythm began immediately as I hit the ground running and tried to get some sense of what was going on around me. After a week of trying to pull things into a straight line I met Janey, the freelance writer. She was in her early thirties, attractive and obviously intelligent but had a sassy tongue and I can remember thinking to myself, 'You're going to have to go, lady', but how wrong I was on that score, as it transpired.

If you've ever seen the eighties sitcom series *WKRP Cincinnati*, about a crazy radio station and its equally crazy staff, you'll know what I mean when I compare what was going on around me to be the newspaper version of that show.

Some days, an agitated creditor would come up the office stairs, yelling about money that Abe owed him to which Abe would cluck away sympathetically and then offer to repay his debt at $5 a week forever, whilst pointedly highlighting the fact that if said agitated creditor put him into bankruptcy, that Abe's first creditor was the Inland Revenue Department, so anyone silly enough to pay the legal bankruptcy fees to put Abe under would get nothing, as the IRD would grab anything that wasn't nailed down as, by law, they automatically were the government guaranteed first creditor.

Because part of my deal for accepting the job was that I had total control over all decision-making, meant that I could get up to speed fairly quickly and in a short space of time I'd managed to resurrect a lot of my old clients from my earlier times at the radio station and convince them that I was intending to build a successful publication but needed their backing to get going in exchange for giving them low-cost advertising rates.

After around 10 days, the first night of paper production commenced with Abe, Janey and myself all hunched over the light tables furiously assembling stories which Abe would invariably paste in the wrong sequence or upside down so that nothing made sense, but it was a laugh a minute. The old days at the 'Na-Na' meetings with the Byron Bay junkies now seemed very far away indeed. It was 3am on that first production night when I got home, flopped into bed and then back to the office at 7am to get things ready for the print deadline.

Any floating anxiety I felt was now based on reality, not on demons from my subconscious rubbish bin, and I started to notice the old juices and neural pathways kicking back in to support me as I assembled new concepts in my mind and brain. What a great feeling! For the first time in over two years, I began to feel alive and vaguely normal again. It seemed as if all the dark days of going to hell and back were peeling into the slipstream of my past and were now justifying my initial decision to kick the benzo habit and swim to the light.

It would be fair to say that getting a fresh challenge in a game you understand is a crucial breakthrough for any recovering addict after going through recovery and the reality was that without this opportunity to 'strut my stuff' it's debatable where I would've ended up. After all, it was only a few weeks back that I'd been unemployed with no future in sight.

If you are addicted or going through withdrawal right now, I would say this to you. You must always hold on to the belief that some sort of higher power or the God of junkies and drag queens in limousines, or whatever, will always be there for you if you don't give up and, as in my case, eventually the clouds of opportunity will peel back revealing blue skies and a hopeful future for you. You must hold that thought until that time comes as you struggle along in your recovery, because it *will* arrive if you stay on track and, until then, just keep batting the demons away one day at a time. If you're totally focused on being drug-free, there are 'angels' there to support you if you don't give up. It may not seem like it on the day but you can make it. I did, which is what this book is about. Hope!

We finished putting that first paper production together and off it went to the printers, which was oddly enough owned by the same company who published the large daily newspaper and technically were our opposition. Prior to my arrival, they had obviously seen Abe's paper as being of such little consequence that they figured they may as well take his money, but therein lies the rub. It turned out that Abe hadn't been paying his printing bills. I received a phone call that afternoon from the general manager of the printers informing me that until a bill for 8K was paid for past printing costs, the current issue wouldn't go to print. Given I'd sweated my backside off convincing old clients to come on board and all the late-night labour that had gone into production, I couldn't let this happen.

From memory, I had about 12K left in my bank account and thinking that it was too late to turn back now in this movie called *Rob's New Job*, I dug into my account, paid the outstanding bills with a lien on future advertising earnings for repayment, and the paper rolled off the press and into the public's letterboxes around the coverage area.

Accentuating the positive, I'd pirated a PR photo of the latest-release Mercedes Benz saloon with two glamorous people admiring the lines of the car. I blew it up to half the front cover of the paper with the caption 'Your local newspaper staff admiring the new company car', with the upshot being we got immediate feedback that the paper must be doing better than it appeared to be. We were up and running and ready for the madness that ensued.

36

Romance and little critters

As mentioned earlier, one of the edicts and rules of Narcotics Anonymous is that you should not enter into any emotional or romantic relationships for at least two years after your recovery commences, for the obvious reason that if things fall apart due to your emotional fragility and fledgling recovery, your first thought would be pick up the drugs (or alcohol) again to numb the pain as you'd always done in the past.

No romantic opportunities like that had presented themselves to me during recovery in Australia, other than that of a casual nature with a couple of hippie chicks back in Byron Bay, one of whom had skilled me up on the supposed joys of Tantric sex and the dubious merits of delayed orgasms.

But now that I was gainfully employed, like everything else around me, the momentum in my life built up speed at a fast pace. The smart-tongued freelance writer, Janey, started showing obvious signs of flirtation, much to the amusement of the others around us, and soon we were having a great old time together.

She was excellent fun, initially, and an extremely good writer, so we made a dynamic combo at work. Without her input, I'm not quite sure how things would've panned out, but that's totally subjective as she was also very temperamental to manage and there were many volatile incidents, which bordered on me telling her to go well before the eventual end of the relationship five years later. I think that old adage about not working with someone that you're romantically involved with is very true, as it's hard to be a boss, a colleague and a lover without hitting speed bumps. It becomes really apparent how things can change when you split up and are still working together, which is exactly how it turned out for me.

Outside of the work environment our life was great. When we hooked up, Janey had two young children, so over the next few years that we were all together, we had a wonderful time picnicking around the countryside on the weekends, tucking the children into bed at night, reading them stories and doing all the things normal people do.

I will always be grateful to her for giving me that invaluable experience of herself and the children and including me as an integral part of a semi-nuclear family unit for those precious few years.

Meanwhile, back in the jungle, the popularity of the paper grew at a rapid pace. Within a couple of years, we were the toast of the 'great white set'. Janey and I were invited to prestige functions, winery launches and lived like royalty on free lunches and her fine dinners, which were as good as anything Jamie Oliver could conjure up.

Throughout all the earlier years of taking pills, recovery and my breakthrough into the newspaper and relationship scene with Janey, I always nursed a feeling of somehow being 'weak' for taking pills and an associated sense of guilt.

It's taken me a very long time to overcome this way of thinking and I know most of you reading this will relate to that feeling if you've been addicted.

I never told her or, for that matter, anyone in subsequent relationships or even close friends about what I perceived to be my 'horrible little secret'. The only other comparison I can make is the crushing feeling of guilt and failure that I also experienced when my marriage broke up and again this reaction is apparently very normal and typical. I sometimes wonder whether it wasn't the fallout from my marriage break-up that activated those first, powerful feelings of anxiety in me and led me to taking my initial lot of benzos? This is largely why it's taken me so long to write this book, as I didn't want anyone I knew to find out about what I perceived as my 'secret weakness', and even up until my most recent relationship, I've never spoken about my dark days of addiction. Writing this book is my kiss goodbye to the past and any feelings of shame or inadequacy.

It has been very cathartic for me. I'm now at such a strong position in my life that other people's opinions are of very little concern to me, as I am a free man in all ways and not dependent on other humans for my state of wellbeing.

37

Fortune, fame and The Golden Dawn

The months rolled on by, as did the fortnightly newspapers off the printing presses, and accordingly my life prospered in all ways. I had modelled the style of my paper on one that I used to read back in Byron Bay during the recovery daze called *The Echo*, which had an irreverent attitude to corporates, snowflakes and political tossers, and its zany style translated well into my own publication.

It soon became a 'must read' to the targeted public and it was accepted into the collective consciousness of the local community as 'their paper'. Even though I was still suffering from daily anxiety over and above what you would call normal levels, I seemed to have picked up a new rhythm of acceptance of the fact that 'some days were going to be diamonds, and some days were going to be stones' and roll with whatever my brain and psychology delivered to me, as it was out of my control either way.

Unfortunately, on those days when the brain chemistry wasn't delivering the right, natural anti-anxiety brain chemicals to the GABA receptors, I would feel anxiety levels completely out of proportion to what was actually going on around me and even hypothetically winning the Lottery would still not relieve it, but next day it would be gone like the rain after the storm, with no rhyme or reason as to what had stressed me the previous day. These days still occasionally continue to appear from nowhere but that's part of the fallout from the earlier years and I just roll with it. There were many times I'd tell the office that I had to see a client when, in reality, I would head to the peace and quiet of my little home by the swimming pool to do some meditation and rebalance my mind.

New Zealanders will know Havelock North, where I lived, as being what Buckinghamshire is to London or the Hamptons are to New York. In other words, it was at the top of the affluence tribal dial and where those rich people live with all the dosh. There were statistically more BMWs and Audis per head of population in Havelock North than anywhere else in New Zealand, so I'm sure you get my drift. For me, having been to an expensive boarding school as a child and coming from a reasonably well-off background, it was easy to understand the tolerance levels and the inverted humour of my newspaper target audience and I went for it like a heat-seeking missile, hitting the target every time.

We catered to the polo set, the upmarket private girls' and boys' schools in the area. We ran features on wineries in the region's version of Napa Valley, 'The Great Chefs of The Bay', fashion features, etc., plastering the paper with flattering photos of the local caricatures of the Kardashians, whilst catering to grassroots activities at schools and local sport clubs.

All the while, nobody knew anything about what I'd been through in my recovery from prescription pills in Australia. My back story was that I had been a successful radio personality (which was true) who had been away overseas for the last few years, so you can imagine my secret smile when I'd find myself writing a character reference for a local cop or having a coffee in my office with the Mayor or a local politician. In amongst them there were some really good people and genuine characters, but whatever we were doing with the paper, it really worked.

You may have noticed that I now refer to it as 'my' newspaper. That's because after about 18 months from the start of my time at the paper, I had managed to bring in a large amount of advertising revenue, increase the page count, turn a profit and get a good buzz of acceptance amongst the readers in our delivery area, which was Havelock North along with upper sociographic environs elsewhere around Hawke's Bay. Unfortunately, my business partner, Abe, despite doing his best, was not able to effectively contribute technically and most of the time probably only knew what the paper was doing when he read it after each publication hit the streets. He was a lovely man and a genuine soul but given the paper was nearly dead when I met him, it was obvious he wasn't quite up to handling what was now a rapidly developing business as the paper continued to grow in popularity and, accordingly, so did the work input requirements. So, I bought out his shareholding and we took a quantum leap forward.

I was now starting to make serious money, a lot of which

I ploughed back into the business, hiring more and better staff and installing the latest publishing technology. Within three years from starting at the paper, I had moved from my rented, poolside haven and put down a mortgage on my own house, which I paid off in 18 months.

It's very hard to not believe in magic when you're living in your own home, yet only less than five years back I was a shivering mess, nursing a recovery from benzo tranquilliser addiction, whilst holed up in an upstairs loft in a beach town in Australia, with nothing to my name but a few possessions, a second-hand car and a meagre number of bucks in the bank.

But when the brass ring comes around for what I perceived as the last time for me, as I wasn't getting any younger, you grasp it in both hands and, as Jason Isbell would say, you go for it, doing all the hard yards required to set yourself free forever, which is exactly what I did. Thank you, Higher Power!

There's an interesting sidebar to this saga of Havelock North, the whole newspaper thing and me. Havelock North had a curious history of eccentrics and philosophers and subscribers to the alternative, esoteric and occult ways of thinking embedded amongst its population.

My mother had married (for the second time) a lovely, older gentleman in the truest sense of the word, who had been a member of the illustrious and ancient Hermetic Order of the Golden Dawn (Stella Matutina), which had been re-ignited in Havelock North as its centre, after all its members had fled London when the 'wickedest man on earth' Aleister 'The Beast' Crowley infiltrated the Dawn's ranks, learnt their secret rituals and then proceeded to print them for all and sundry to access.

The ultimate ambition of the Golden Dawn's adepts was to utilise the 'magical imagination' — a process which involved 'visualising a desired reality', concentrating one's will on it, 'moulding its form in astral light' and bringing it, finally, into 'the plainest physical reality'.

Under the leadership of a charismatic Englishman called Dr Felkin, most of the fleeing Golden Dawn members in the UK washed up in Havelock North and immediately built a fascinating Chapman-Taylor architecturally designed house with a large, secret crypt below which was covered in Egyptian hieroglyphics on the walls for the purpose of worshipping the occult and specifically the Sun God, Ra, with the ultimate intention of manifesting the second coming of the Christ Force. Because of my relationship with my stepfather, I already knew quite a lot about the undercurrent of the Havelock North history before I ever started at the paper, not only on the surface of the local 'rich and famous' but of the historical past of the intelligentsia who were the local equivalent of the famous English Bloomsbury set. In the mid-1920s, New Zealanders had also awoken to discover that everyone in high places, from Governor-General to Chief Justice, Prime Minister to Police Commissioner, was a Magister Templi in Havelock North's occult society of The Golden Dawn.

You may wonder why I mention this.

It honestly seemed to me that the turnaround in my life had been so spectacular, from zero to hero, that I always had this strange feeling that when the paper appeared out of nowhere at a very low point in my life, offering me a golden opportunity to save myself from an extremely bleak, future existence, that the whole thing had been overseen by something greater than me, testing to see whether I had learnt my karmic life lessons in my days of drug recovery.

Like, what would I do with my new-found freedom from pills and would I squander the opportunity being given to me to build a good life again?

That probably sounds like mumbo-jumbo to the average person, but I suspect those of you who have bought my book have bought it in an effort to find some clues as to how to set your own self free from addictive substances and can relate to my belief system at that time. You must have something to believe in when you're struggling to be free, and taking comfort from the invisible can be a trusty ally.

I chose to believe and genuinely still feel, to this very day, that the Fates were on my side if I tried my best in the material world. To that end, I often embedded in the text of the paper messages of an esoteric or positive nature that only a certain school of thought would understand. I was paying back my dues for the good luck that now seemed to surround me after my dark days in the past.

I can remember thinking at the time that the gods don't give you rewards unless you show you're capable of handling them. Whatever the truth was, it worked for me to believe this way of looking at my life.

38

——

The big payoff

Based on the whole newspaper saga appearing in my life as if from nowhere, I also came to be thinking that the 'gift' had a limited life and the trick was not to stay too long at the 'fair' simply making money and running a local paper. So, I slowly formulated in my mind an exit strategy to sell and move on to my next step into the unknown.

Maybe the ghosts of the long-departed good ol' boys from the Golden Dawn were still hovering in the local ether and some stray Na-Nas etc. were telepathically watching me from Byron Bay to see whether I'd been seduced by the good money and the cool life I was now leading. Had I made the fatal mistake of becoming just another parody of my former, immature self or would I be smart and take the plunge into the next frame of my life's movie? This was my test as I saw it at that time.

Because I had grown the paper to be very successful with

capable staff and a very good income stream, it was now a desirable asset, so I set up a plan to play my paper off against the other two major corporate-owned newspapers in the region, in an endeavour to extract the highest possible value upon sale.

For the last three years, before I eventually sold, I was personally earning nett NZ$180,000 annually, so you can see that it was a bit of a challenge to walk away from that steady income stream and rising, but I did.

It may seem like I'd gone from suffering through withdrawal in the early days to a sudden Walt Disney-type fairy-tale ending to my circumstances, but I can assure you that it wasn't simply a cakewalk as soon as I started the uphill trek from my beginnings at the newspaper. There were many, many highs and lows but there's no point in dwelling on the negatives that naturally occurred. By now, I'd owned the paper for nine amazing years. My state of mind and neural pathways were as good as they were ever going to get, considering the past. I was no different to the next person in the madhouse of everyday life except that I now owned a home, a good car and was financially secure.

My original plan upon leaving Byron Bay and limping back to New Zealand nearly 10 years earlier to slowly rebuild my life and a personal sense of worth had been achieved to the best of my ability and it was time to insert a new Rob Pharazyn personal DVD into the Blu-ray slot and see what life would offer me next.

I was only in my early fifties and there was a lot of the world to see, fun to be had and life to be lived. My relationship with Janey had ended in a rather unpleasant way, so I was single, fancy-free and soon to be very cashed up.

I drew up a letter to the management of APN Newspapers NZ, who were owned (amongst many other media outlets, globally) by Tony O'Reilly, the billionaire Irishman. I was in a very good bargaining position, as my paper was powering along, earning great money from regional and national advertising, and I was circled like a lone Red Indian by the 'wagons' of the two main corporate print conglomerates of APN and Fairfax of Australia, whose daily papers competed in the same region as me.

On my slow run-up to offering the paper for sale, my next move was to go to the most powerful stockbroking firm in town, which was headed by a respected local businessman, who was a fan of my paper. I asked him if he would be willing to be my front man or go-between to get into negotiations with either of the aforementioned corporates. He gladly agreed, so my first shot across the bows went out to APN head office in Auckland City on the gold–embossed letterhead of the stockbrokers and it was game on!

As in my earlier chapters of the weird stories related to my time of hanging out with the NA crew in my early recovery in Byron Bay, it's tempting to recount the fun and games that took place between myself and APN as we jostled them into place to get a maximum result, but the main thrust of this book is to give hope to recovering addicts, so I'll stick to the point, because I was about to be rewarded in spectacular fashion!

The big day arrived for negotiating the sale and the head of APN New Zealand flew into town with his 'yes' men. Along with the management of their local daily paper, myself and Barron (the head of the stockbroking firm) all assembled in the hallowed boardroom, with the heavy, gilt-framed photos of the chairmen and stockbrokers of a hundred years past silently looking down on the proceedings.

In my opinion, the trick of going into any big negotiation is to have the mindset that you don't mind if it doesn't succeed, as you then have a clear picture of what you want to achieve and if that doesn't happen then there's always tomorrow. The procedure when you sell a prosperous business is that you start negotiation with what's known as a multiple figure, which is simplistically a multiplied equation of annual nett earnings against overheads, etc.

Our plan was to come in from the high ground and make their eyes water early in the piece, so we passed over a multiple asking price for my paper of NZ$1.3 million. They looked at it, gulped and muttered something along the lines of 'no way will we pay that', so I stood up and said, 'Oh well, that's that. Time to get back to work' and started packing up my briefcase, which had the desired effect. They asked for time to discuss things, so Barron and I went to another part of the building, drank tea and waited. Within 30 minutes they reappeared and handed over the original document we'd presented asking for $1.3 million. They had scratched out that asking figure, putting in their countersigned offer of $500,000!

Considering my paper came out only fortnightly, was free to the public, totally reliant on advertising and the actual goods and chattels as part of the sale were a few desks, computers and tech gear valued at NZ$15,000; half a million bucks wasn't too bad, you would think?

Once upon a time in my teenage years, I'd spent five months living off playing stud poker, which had paid my weekly rent, etc. and included winning a Volkswagen car off a Yank who worked at the American Embassy, so you could say raising the odds was in my blood. I reached over and scrawled out their NZ$500,000 offer and wrote a counter offer of $550,000, plus I was to also keep the final audit trail of debts outstanding to 90 days that amounted to another 50K, which took my price of acceptance to NZ$600,000. It was a Tuesday, so the final kicker was that my offer was only on the table till 11am the coming Friday morning, giving them just under three days to make up their minds. That was it. We all shook hands and went our separate ways.

It was a lovely sunny spring afternoon as I left the building in a kind of a daze and stepped out onto the busy street. I drove out to a beautiful beach on the coast and deliriously threw my hands to the sky and, yelling like a banshee, thanked every deity known to mankind for this wonderful result. What a feeling it was on that day, what a joyous moment to behold! After all the trials and tribulations I had been through over the past decade, to now be financially free. Fortune favours the brave and until you take that first step onto the 1000-mile rice paper, grasshopper, you are never going to get anywhere.

Friday morning came around and right on the stroke of 11am, my mobile phone rang and the head of APN for the South Pacific informed me that he would accept my deal and congratulated me on driving a good bargain.

Now, you'd be forgiven for thinking that all I had to do now was to bank the money, but it's not that simple. When you sell a business, as I had done, all that was in place at this point was that both parties had signed an agreement to the purchase price, goods and chattels, etc. in what is known as a 'memorandum of understanding', but it wasn't the end of negotiations. They then have the right to do what's called 'due diligence', which basically means they can then get their accountants and lawyers to start trying to find reasons why they shouldn't pay the full agreed price because of some minuscule detail. In other words, try to beat you down to accepting less than the original offer. They played their silly game for about two months until I got tired of it and fired off a memo telling them that I was withdrawing the paper from sale unless the deal went through pronto and fully intact, as first agreed.

Within days, one of their money people flew in, wined and dined me, talked to my accountants and all was signed, sealed and delivered for full payment to be made to me on 15 December 2001. (Just in time to be the biggest Christmas present I'd ever had!) Came the 15th and, at the prearranged time of 3pm, I sat looking at the online balance on my laptop computer of the amount in the company bank account. Suddenly, the numbers $550,000 appeared and booted the balance to well above the half-million-dollar mark!

More magic, but now it was real.

I had made it to freedom and, unless I acted stupidly and went out and bought fast cars and boats, I would be fairly well set up for my future as a newly-born millionaire. Well done, give that man a Mars bar!

39

Roaming the world after recovery

I trust you're all still with me and enjoying the success I had scored after wading my way through the muck of recovery from benzos, because what I'm trying to convey to you is that there can be a pot of gold at the end of the rainbow if you'll just make the initial start to bite the bullet and get off whatever drug you're on.

Christmas came and went and as the year rolled over into 2002, I got busy setting myself up for my next move, which was to hit the deck running and travel, travel, travel and that is exactly what I did. Like most people, I harboured this fantasy of being the intrepid traveller burdened with nothing but a backpack, credit card and the world as my future playground, so I went to the nearest sports store and bought an expensive and very large backpack with all the bells and whistles needed to climb to the top of Mt Everest or, at the very least, hike along the Amazon with the Jivaro Indians and their poisonous blowpipes. Of course, the reality didn't match the dream, which I soon discovered when I got off the plane into 40-degree heat and 100% humidity at my first big destination, Phuket, in the Land of Smiles, Thailand.

My friends had all waved me goodbye from the airport in New Zealand on the assumption that I was to be gone for months, trekking around South-East Asia as I discovered my 'inner hippie', but after a few days trudging about on Phuket, I came to the conclusion that I wasn't cut out to be a hippie backpacker in the mind-sapping heat, so I checked out of the flea-hole I had booked into online and soon found myself ensconced in something more upmarket near Kata Beach on the other side of the island.

Air-conditioning, swimming at the beach or hotel pool under the tropical sun, sipping on a freshly cut coconut and nights lolling around the Ska Bar set into the cliff off the beach, slurping up Long Island tea cocktails, soon had me getting into the groove of my new lifestyle.

Thailand offers you everything from the department of pleasure which allows you to delude yourself into thinking that you are a very amazing and sexually attractive person, when the reality is usually to the contrary, but although I didn't dip into the honey jar of lithe, young Thai girls pestering me like seagulls at the beach when you're eating fish 'n' chips, the cruise mode gave me my first break in the mental traffic that had been throwing me around like a rag doll for the last decade of recovery, achievement and saying 'adios' to my newspaper business. Whilst lazing on the golden sands of Thailand's beaches, I decided the best course of action into my future was to not have a course of action and to just go for it, with travel to exotic far-flung parts of the world, which is exactly what I did. After charging my batteries in Thailand, I returned home to the jibes from my friends about my sudden reappearance after just a few weeks, but it was all in good fun.

Over the next four years, I managed to get into a great relationship with a gorgeous woman nearly half my age, who had a loving heart and a libido like the Witch Queen of New Orleans and together we bounced around in Egypt, Jordan (Petra), Thailand and Bali for three months and then, leaving her back in New Zealand, I took off again roaming around the world until 2006. The United States (I slid through New Orleans three weeks before Katrina hit), Greek islands, UK, France, Italy, Morocco, Borneo, Turkey and on and on it went through different countries, sailing, trekking, swimming, carousing about until I really had put my days of being a recovering addict and businessman well and truly into my past.

40

Was it all worth it?

One of the ironies of life is that everywhere you go you take the weather with you, and the constant, bloody anxiety and repetitive over-thinking that had haunted me for years still sat on my shoulder like a vindictive parrot, persecuting me with unnecessary thoughts, making enjoyment harder to achieve in living my new lifestyle, but generally it would've been ungrateful of me to be moaning. As they say, money can't buy you happiness, which is true, but I'm here to tell you that it sure as hell buys you a far better brand of unhappiness and ranks right up there with oxygen!

I had come to accept that post-recovery from benzo addiction, a sense of simmering anxiety beyond my control would remain with me, rearing its ugly head on certain days for the rest of my life, although nowadays my life seems to be serene and only occasionally do I have an inexplicably anxiety-riven day!

The receptors in my brain are, unfortunately, never ever again going to quite rewire back to what they were before my chemical dependency on Ativan and, like being killed in a firefight in Syria, this is simply what is known as 'collateral damage' and I knew that this was something that I would just have to live with throughout my life, regardless of how much travelling I did or pleasurable activities I got into.

The stark reality is that after going through so much trauma and basically near-death experiences as you battle suicidal ideation and abject misery during the withdrawal and recovery process, you obviously can never be the same person ever again and the mental and emotional scars will always be with you, so you just have to get used to it.

Never being the person you once were, pre-detox, may not necessarily be a bad thing, as look at the mess it got you into? You've now evaporated your past and become a different person than the one you knew back in the pre-benzo days, so enjoy it and keep going forward. To me, it's a small price to pay for freedom from a drug that had controlled my very being for 13 years and forced me to bend to its will as it demanded its daily fix. I have always said that no matter what your drug of choice is, as long as it is revolving around you and you are in control of your intake, then you are comparatively safe, as some weekend heroin users will attest to, but I'm also here to tell you that that can never happen with benzos as, once you start down the road of benzodiazepines, within weeks you are addicted and unless you are given early advice, you will end up revolving around your daily pills like a lonely little satellite, lost in orbit.

It would've been easy for me to feel sorry for myself for the price I'd had to pay through no fault of my own after taking something prescribed by a medical professional, but what was the point? What's done is done and was all just part of the ongoing movie known as my life. So, I just copped the mental fallout as part of the deal and worked on mitigating it with meditation, etc. and counting my current blessings. The Buddha said, 'Suffering is resistance to what *is*' and in my case what *is* was that I'd been to a chemical hell and back and survived.

For me it was Ativan but in your world, it may be any one of the non-benzo drugs prescribed by the medical profession such as Oxy, Trammies, Zops or Vicodin, etc. or, for that matter, it could be cocaine, smack, meth, alcohol, you name it — it's all there to shore up your fragile mental ecosystem as you dampen down the inner hysteria, trying to stay sane and still be part of everyday life. What most of us don't realise is that everybody, and I mean everybody, that you pass in the street, see on the television or whatever, are *all* in the same mad lifeboat and are just trying to shut down that monkey mind leaping from branch to branch inside their head. Just because they're smiling doesn't mean they're happy!

So how do I wrap this story up?

After around four years of consistent global travel, I came back to Havelock North where I had lived and been so richly rewarded by the owning of a newspaper. I sold up my home, moving north of Auckland City, New Zealand, hanging out for five years at a beautiful beach where I rented a townhouse by the ocean, bought a boat and went fishing. I did some talkback radio but only enough to confirm to myself that it was now more toxic than what I'd left behind some years back, and for the rest of my time in the north, I just grooved around the beach and spent days in the city going to concerts, sitting on busy streets watching cute, young Japanese girls and feeling pity for the stressed-out office people. I had a couple of unfortunate experiences beyond my control (one of which nearly cost me my eyesight), before deciding it was time to head back south to Havelock North to fulfil a long-held dream, which was to get a dog, buy a special type of house and just kick back and let the world slide on by.

I'd done enough to fill 10 lives and, like Voltaire's Candide, I was planning to be content to just sit around and listen to loud music, read books and wear my Hawaiian shirts whilst drinking tequila at sunset, blissfully ignoring the outside world. It didn't quite work out like that as my roguish nature made sure that I still got up to mischief, but now, here I am, in my Laurel Canyon-style mansion surrounded by beautiful bush at the top of a tree-lined driveway. Do the gods reward you if you give it a go to clean up your life? It seems that they do! My house is three storeys, with an elevator running from the downstairs garage up to the internal hallway, a deck that wraps around the exterior of the whole inner living area, with a view across the plains to the mountains which, in winter, get snowcapped so when I'm on the top floor lying in my bed, I don't even have to raise my head off the pillow to take in all the beauty and blue skies.

I would be lying if I didn't say that it would be great to put the icing on the cake and have a good woman to share all this with, but again it's that collateral damage thing.

After all I've been through, I think I've become gun-shy about anything involving giving too much of myself, when the 'myself' is something I've nearly lost so many times in the torrent I was caught up in in the past.

Ships in the night come (literally) and go but it would take a special kind of person to synch into where my head is at, but you never say never? I'm just grateful that I made it to the 'shore' and that 'the horror, the horror', as Colonel Kurtz would say, is finally over. I have found my Ithaca and am at peace with myself.

41

The last hurrah

On November the 14th, 2016, I went back.

The last NA meeting I'd attended was in the early nineties but here I was now, waiting outside the Masonic Hall, Byron Bay, for the usual, scheduled 7.30pm Friday night meeting of the 'Na-Nas', with the only difference being that I was now no longer suffering as a recovering benzo addict.

The location had changed from the old Byron Bay community centre but the reality is that some things in the twilight world of drugs, junkies and recovery never change, except it was now 24 years and a lifetime later and returning to the 'scene of the crime' seemed a fitting end to the saga of my past life and this book.

It was a lovely, golden-syrupy, tropical evening as the sun headed into the west.

I parked my rental car under a tall palm tree in the car park opposite the hall and waited for them to come. The usual bronzed tourists were scuttling around the streets get-ting ready to glide into the heart of Friday night for some sex, drugs and rock'n'roll mayhem around Byron Bay, whilst on the other side of the tracks the damaged were somewhere nearby and heading to their usual Friday night Narcotics Anonymous lifeline. As the minutes ticked down towards 7.30pm, there was no sign of anybody except for a small woman who had appeared and proceeded to unlock the main doors to the hall.

My original intention was to return to my past and attend this meeting to recount my story of what had happened to me since I'd last been there all those years ago, in the hope that my tale may provide some inspiration, but deep down I knew that it would be seen as bragging, having seen the same shining examples at meetings back in the day and scoffed at their braggadocio.

Seven-thirty ticked over and still no one had shown, then slowly like silent spectres they came, materialising out of the dusk from shop alleys and seemingly from nowhere. First one man and then two girls and then a small assortment, including a woman who looked in her seventies, continued to manifest, as if out of thin air, and assemble themselves on the ledge outside the Masonic Hall.

A deep sadness swept over me as I recognised Brother Red, Axel and all the rest of the old crew from my past, except it wasn't them any more! It was just replicas of those past comrades and ghosts, still trapped in addiction but in different bodies as they shuffled around doing the manda-tory NA greeting hug whilst all furiously smoking the cheap roll-your-own smokes (can't get rid of all those addictions, can we!).

After about 15 minutes and a few more stragglers later, they slowly shuffled into the hall to hang on to the only sense of reality on offer in their struggle to save themselves one more time. Just as the last one disappeared inside, a large motorbike pulled up beside me and a big, burly man, covered in tatts, ripped off his crash helmet and gave me the usual 'G'day, mate' greeting through my lowered car window. I responded in kind and then he said, 'Well, time to head off to the right place for me' as he walked towards the hall.

As he strode away, I leant out the car window and called out, 'Say hi to the Na-Nas for me', which stopped him in his tracks. Only an ex-Byron Bay Na-Na would know that that was the code name used back then by each other for all the fallen angels.

He turned and smiled, gave me a thumbs up and with that he disappeared into the Friday night meeting.

Let the storm come. For after the storm comes the rainbow. I booted up the car engine and drove away, knowing in my heart and soul that I had ticked the last box.

It was over...

PART IV

The Facts

42

Background information

After going through the nightmare of withdrawal and recovery, it may not seem like it at the time but your addiction has probably given you a second chance and a golden opportunity to change your life. Obviously, you can't continue acting as you did during the taking of prescription drugs like benzos (or any recreational drugs, for that matter) because the whole purpose of giving up an addiction is to live a better, brighter, more fulfilling life.

Recovery is difficult not just because of the detox and withdrawal tapering process but because you have to change your life and all change is difficult, even under general circumstances.

If you use this opportunity for change, you'll look back and think of your addiction as maybe one of the best things that ever happened to you. People in recovery often describe themselves as grateful addicts. Why would someone be grateful to have survived an addiction, you may ask?

Because through the sometimes life-threatening process of shedding their addiction, recovered addicts often find an inner peace and tranquillity that most people crave but can never seem to find.

I personally know that you can't go into the abyss, as I did, and experience the threatening of your very existence without emerging as a different person.

So how did it all come to this?

In this modern world, it's easy to find a 'crutch' to help you through the madness, but nothing in life ever comes entirely free and invariably 'the bill' arrives asking you to pay for the use of that alcohol, drug, pill or whatever buffer you choose to get you through the day.

Benzodiazepines, including tranquillisers such as Ativan, Xanax, and Valium, and sleeping pills such as Zopiclone, Dalmane, etc — the list goes on — are the bestselling drugs in the history of medicine, with an annual worldwide sales turnover conservatively estimated to be exceeding US$21 billion.

According to my best research, they are prescribed to 30% of the world's population, with two-thirds of those prescriptions going to women. Millions of ongoing repeat prescriptions are written globally, every day, despite medical guidelines for short-term usage of two to four weeks being established and made known to the medical profession over 50 years ago.

Yes, doctors continue to prescribe benzos, despite the known and often serious physical, cognitive and crippling emotional side effects. It beggars belief that this behaviour continues to this very day, but it does and here's why. The short answer is, naturally, the money-go-round. It's a reasonably well-known fact that, generally speaking, the big pharmaceutical drug companies market their products onto doctors with one purpose, which is to make money for their shareholders.

The pharmaceutical industry is vastly wealthy. By 2014, it had reached the US$1 trillion mark. That is a staggering amount of money. An industry that rich can afford to spend significant amounts of money in courting political influence. The magnitude of the pharmaceutical industry's investment is considerable; from political lobbying, right down to the medical rep calling on your local doctor offering trips overseas, gifts, etc. for prescribing the drug companies' latest drug du jour.

As they say, drugs are big business.

43

———

Emeritus Professor Heather Ashton

It is now time to introduce Emeritus Professor Heather Ashton into the equation. Professor Ashton is the author of more than 50 published papers about benzodiazepine drugs. Holding multiple degrees in Medicine from the University of Oxford, she became a Member of the Royal College of Physicians in 1958, and a Fellow of the Royal College of Physicians in 1975.

She has served as National Health Service Consultant in both Clinical Psychopharmacology and Psychiatry. Now 88 years of age, in failing health and retired as Emeritus Professor of Clinical Psychopharmacology at the University of Newcastle upon Tyne, in Britain, her research at the university focused on the nature of psychotropic drugs and their effects upon the brain and upon behaviour.

She operated a benzodiazepine withdrawal clinic for 12 years in England, and has provided expert testimony about benzodiazepines in both governmental investigations as well as courtroom litigations.

Therefore, she is arguably the world's foremost expert on these drugs, and her book and papers entitled *Benzodiazepines: How They Work and How to Withdraw* would have to be recognised as the gold standard of information if you were seeking to proceed towards ridding yourself of any of the benzodiazepine group of drugs.

Links to her website and all you'll need to know are a few pages further on in this section of the book. Also, here is a link to a multitude of testimonials from benzo dependent people who found the works of Professor Ashton extremely beneficial in their quest to be free from addiction. http://www.recovery-road.org/prof-ashtons-work. To some recovered addicts, Heather Ashton is an angel who saved their life.

I am very fortunate, grateful (and flattered) to be recognised by Professor Ashton in my endeavours to bring this book to the global public and benzo-dependent sufferers by having her permission to use any of her research material, so the following section of this book is based on the researched advice gained over the years by Professor Ashton and outlined in her acclaimed work, *The Ashton Manual*.

After much digging, I located her to ask for that permission but, sadly, she was nearly at the end of her rewarding life. I received this email from her son in the UK on 30 January 2017.

Dear Rob

I'm afraid my mother is seriously ill. She will not recover, and is unable to deal with correspondence. But I have read your message to her.

Too many people continue to suffer under the scourge of benzo dependency. And too many find it hard to see the light at the end of the tunnel. My mother always urges those who manage to find it to tell their story, as a beacon for everyone else.

So, she is delighted you are doing that. She would be content for you to quote from her published work, including the Ashton Manual, providing you do so without editing and verbatim, and you point readers towards the original texts so that the passages you use can easily be put in context. You might also point out to readers that my mother has never sought to secure commercial benefit from her work, shunning all offers to do so.

I hope that is helpful. Good luck with your writing

John Ashton

Thank you, John! In her own words, here is Heather's overview of the benzo scourge.

For twelve years (1982–1994) I ran a Benzodiazepine Withdrawal Clinic in the UK for people wanting to come off their tranquillisers and sleeping pills.

Much of what I know about this subject was taught to me by those brave and long-suffering men and women. By listening to the histories of over 300 'patients' and by closely following their progress (week-by-week and sometimes day-by-day), I gradually learned what long-term benzodiazepine use and subsequent withdrawal entails.

Most of the people attending the clinic had been taking benzodiazepines prescribed by their doctors for many years, sometimes over 20 years. They wished to stop because they did not feel well.

They realised that the drugs, though effective when first prescribed, might be actually making them feel ill.

They had many symptoms, both physical and mental. Some were depressed and/or anxious; some had 'irritable bowel', cardiac or neurological complaints. Many had undergone hospital investigations with full gastrointestinal, cardiological and neurological screens (nearly always with negative results). A number had been told (wrongly) that they had multiple sclerosis. Several had lost their jobs through recurrent illnesses.

The experiences of these patients have since been confirmed in many studies, by thousands of patients attending tranquilliser support groups in the UK and other parts of Europe, and by individuals vainly seeking help in the US. It is interesting that the patients themselves, and not the medical profession, were the first to realise that long-term use of benzodiazepines could cause problems.

— Emeritus Professor Heather Ashton

44

Why should you come off
benzodiazepines?

There are many reasons why you should come off benzos, but the main one is that they would've probably only been effective for the first few months that you started taking them and now, in my experience, they are simply making you feel ill and corroding your soul. Also, long-term use of benzodiazepines can give rise to many unwanted side effects, including poor memory and cognition, emotional blunting, depression, increasing anxiety, physical symptoms and, of course, neurological dependence. It's also worth noting that all benzodiazepines can potentially produce these effects, whether taken as sleeping pills or anti-anxiety drugs.

They lose much of their efficacy very quickly because of the development of tolerance. When tolerance develops, unrecognised 'withdrawal' symptoms can appear, even though the user continues to take the drug, unaware that they're effectively constantly in withdrawal due to the nature of the drug which is what happened to me owing to the short half-life of the Ativan I was on.

Thus, the symptoms suffered by many long-term users are a mixture of adverse effects of the drugs and 'withdrawal' effects due to built-up tolerance.

Many users, such as myself, have remarked that it was not until after they came off their drugs that they realised they had been operating in their everyday life at a level well below par, for all the years they had been taking the benzo pre-scribed to them.

When I finally put adequate time between my initial detox and full recovery, for me it was as though a curtain or veil had been pulled back in my life revealing brighter colours, more energy, better sleep and happier state of mind. In short, a brand-new world that seemed like what I recalled from my younger days. Who wouldn't want that?

A lot of 'withdrawal symptoms' are not necessarily phys-ical or mental symptoms but simply due to fear of with-drawal (or even fear of that fear). As the old saying goes, 'the only thing to fear is fear itself'.

People who have had bad experiences when having a go at giving up their daily benzo have usually been withdraw-ing too quickly without being given any decent explanation of the expected symptoms. Consequently, they don't want to go back into that initial burst of symptoms that accompany the early stages of withdrawal, so they retreat back onto the pills, which makes them continue to live a half-life of numb-ness.

Take no notice of any doctor or shrink who tells you to

just stop taking your pills and go 'cold turkey' without first seeking advice about a planned programme of slow withdrawal. That path leads to dangerous outcomes.

It may bring comfort to those contemplating ceasing taking benzos to know that, at the other extreme, some people can stop their benzodiazepines with absolutely no symptoms at all, but I would say that that would be the exception to the rule. The easy answer is to seek and take advice and then start off slowly. You'll soon find out how you will react, but try to avoid being obsessive and focusing, minute by minute, on how you're feeling emotionally and physically as you enter withdrawal. Hard to do, I know, but it will serve no useful purpose to over-think the process.

Nobody should be forced or persuaded to withdraw against his or her will. Anecdotal evidence suggests that people who are unwillingly pushed into withdrawal often do badly. On the other hand, the chances of success are very high for those who are sufficiently motivated. Anyone who really wants to come off, can come off benzodiazepines. I'm living proof that it can be done. The choice is entirely personal, but everyone deserves a second chance at life and this can be yours.

45

Before starting benzo withdrawal

The option, the choice and therefore the decision is one that any user of benzodiazepines should not enter into lightly. They must consider, and consider carefully, and with great deliberation all the parameters before proceeding. Once you have made up your mind to withdraw, there are some steps, as outlined in *The Ashton Manual*, to take before you start.

(1) Firstly, consult your doctor who has been prescribing benzos to you and also the dispensing pharmacist who filled your script. A good preparatory option before visiting your doctor would be to download an online copy of Professor Ashton's *Benzodiazepines: How They Work and How to Withdraw*, plus a copy of her paper 'Reasons for a Diazepam (Valium) Taper' (available at http://www.benzo.org.uk/ashvtaper.htm), and a cover letter for your doctor stating that you wish to go off the drug. These are useful when you first tell

your chosen doctor of your intentions as it clearly outlines what you're preparing to do.

(2) Remain in control of the situation and don't be swayed by your doctor (or any doctor) telling you that it's not a good idea to stop taking the pills (unless you're in a very unstable state of mind and the benzos are keeping you more stable, but even then, you should hopefully have an aim to eventually come off them).

Your chosen doctor's agreement and co-operation is necessary since he/she will be prescribing the medication you'll need, such as Valium (diazepam) to swing over to from your current brand, due to Valium having the longer half–life, as outlined in the withdrawal chart and information (see chapter 46, The withdrawal).

(3) Many doctors are uncertain how to manage benzodiazepine withdrawal and hesitate to undertake it. But you can reassure your doctor that you intend to oversee your own programme in tandem with him or her and will proceed at whatever pace you find comfortable, although you may value his or her advice from time to time.

Again, it is very important for you to be in control of your own schedule.

The advice in *The Ashton Manual,* which I agree with, is to not let your doctor impose a deadline. It is your mind, body and soul that are going to undergo the withdrawal process and it is imperative that you control the process.

I personally lost my withdrawal control to doctors and shrinks during my early days of uninformed tapering and allowed so-called professionals to prescribe drugs and directions that took me back into a new hell, and only my strength of mind got me back out and on track.

Before you start your programme of detox and withdrawal, sit down and relax. Then at your own pace write down a dosage reduction schedule that you intend to follow.

It can be as slow as you wish but it must have a defined daily and weekly pace. Having a chart that you can follow and make progress marks is necessary to keep giving you a sense of structure in going forward.

Human beings respond better when they have a plan.

As they say, 'fail to plan, plan to fail'. You can amend the plan as you go along if you feel it's too slow or too fast and, as you progress, as you surely will, you may find that you would like to draw up a fresh schedule with different timelines. But always remember that there is no hurry and that you will get to the other end where a happy life awaits you to reward you for your efforts.

(4) Once you have your plan in place and have found your chosen, friendly and preferably holistic doctor who is aware of what you intend to do, make sure you have adequate psychological support. This is extremely important, as to try to go it alone, as I did initially before hooking up with Narcotics Anonymous, is a very challenging task and best to be avoided if possible.

Support could come from your spouse, partner, family or trusted close friend. It's best to have only one reliable person who is totally committed to your wellbeing, as including more people in the mix can often lead to confusion and conflicting advice, which is the last thing you need in your early, fragile stages.

Rather than (or in addition to) expensive therapists, you need someone reliable, who will support you frequently and regularly, long-term, both during withdrawal and for some months or even years afterwards.

Voluntary tranquilliser support groups (self-help groups) can be extremely useful. They are usually run by people who have been through withdrawal and therefore understand the time and patience required and can provide information about benzodiazepines. They can usually be found by searching online for drug support groups in your area.

(5) Get into the right frame of mind.

Now that you've got the basics sorted, it's important that you get into the right frame of mind where you are comfortable with what you are about to undergo — your journey into a clean and brighter future.

If in doubt, try a very small reduction, for a few days, in the dosage of the benzo you're taking (for example, try reducing your daily dosage by about one tenth or one eighth; you may be able to achieve this by halving or quartering one of your tablets).

You will probably find that you notice no difference and this will boost your confidence to go forward. Do not see what you're doing as complete withdrawal in the early stage, even though that is your intention. Anything that eases the burden or unwarranted fear, makes the overall process more acceptable and therefore successful in the end result. You will be surprised to find that you have a strong wish to continue once you have started.

Be patient. There is no need to hurry withdrawal. Your body (and brain) may need time to readjust after years of being on benzodiazepines. Many people have taken a year or more to complete the withdrawal. So, don't rush, and, above all, do not try to suddenly stop taking the benzos.

Choose your own way of approaching things based on information such as what is outlined here — but don't expect a 'quick fix'. The only successful way, based on anecdotal experience, is to follow a programme of researched information from the actual experience of persons who have made it out the other side of addiction, or reliable sources such as *The Ashton Manual*.

Another approach or option may be to enter a hospital or special centre for 'detoxification'. This may suit the busy executive.

Such an approach usually involves quite expensive financial outlay and a rapid withdrawal programme which can be as short as six weeks.

This is medically 'safe' and such clinics may also provide psychological support as part of the package and could be suitable for a small minority of people with difficult psychological problems. However, this often removes the control of withdrawal from the patient and setbacks on returning home are common, largely because there has been no time to build up alternative living skills. Getting clean is not as simple as just going through the physical detox; it's the emotional withdrawal on the other side that is the hardest part.

Clinics can be useful for coming off recreational drugs like smack or meth, but I personally would not recommend using them unless you're a busy 'rock star' or in a desperate (emphasis on desperate) hurry. But it's your call. Once again, you're giving your power away and isn't that what got you into your mess in the first place?

Slow withdrawal in your own environment allows time for physical and psychological adjustments, permits you to continue with your normal life, to tailor your withdrawal to your own lifestyle and to build up alternative strategies for living without benzodiazepines.

It's not just about ridding your bloodstream of a drug. The underlying psychological damage and reasons you were prescribed them in the first place needs to be addressed and that can take a considerable period of time. If these underlying causes aren't worked through, your chances of success are reduced.

46

The withdrawal

1. Dosage tapering

There is absolutely no doubt that anyone withdrawing from long-term benzodiazepines must reduce the dosage slowly and, as I've indicated, I withdrew too quickly, over approximately only four months.

Abrupt or over-rapid withdrawal, especially from high dosages of benzos can give rise to severe symptoms (convulsions, psychotic reactions, acute anxiety states, death, etc.) and may increase the risk of protracted withdrawal symptoms.

Slow withdrawal means tapering your dosage gradually, usually over a period of some months. The aim is to obtain a smooth, steady and slow decline in blood and tissue concentrations of benzodiazepines so that the natural systems in the brain can recover their normal state.

There is scientific evidence that reinstatement of brain function and production of natural GABA takes a long time, and recovery after long-term benzodiazepine use is not unlike the gradual recuperation of the body after a major surgical operation. Healing, of body or mind, is a slow process.

The precise rate of withdrawal is an individual matter. It depends on many factors, including the dose and type of benzodiazepine used, duration of use, personality, lifestyle, previous experience, specific vulnerabilities, and the (perhaps genetically determined) speed of your recovery systems.

Usually the best judge is you, yourself; you must be in control and must proceed at the pace that is comfortable for you.

You may find you need to be firm and resist attempts from outsiders (clinics, doctors) to persuade you into a rapid withdrawal. The classic six weeks withdrawal period adopted by many clinics and doctors is much too fast for many long-term users.

The rate of withdrawal, as long as it is slow enough, is not critical. Whether it takes six months, 12 months or 18 months is of little significance if you have taken benzodiazepines for a matter of years, but the operative word is 'slow'.

It is sometimes claimed that very slow withdrawal from benzodiazepines merely prolongs the agony and it is better to get it over with as quickly as possible. However, the experience of most people is that slow withdrawal is greatly preferable, especially when the person undergoing withdrawal dictates the pace.

Nevertheless, there is no magic rate of withdrawal and each person must find the pace that suits him or her best.

People who have been on low doses of benzodiazepine for a relatively short time (less than a year) can usually withdraw fairly rapidly. Those who have been on very high doses of potent benzodiazepines such as Xanax, Ativan and Klonopin, even for short terms, are likely to need more time.

However, it is important in withdrawal to always be going forwards. If you reach a difficult point, you can have a pit stop there for a few weeks if necessary, but you should try to avoid going backwards and increasing your dosage again.

Some doctors advocate the use of 'escape pills' (an extra dose of benzodiazepines) to be stored for use in particularly stressful situations.

In my experience, this is not sensible advice.

It is not a good idea to take anything more than whatever declining dosage you've achieved in shaving down your pills in your withdrawal progress, as it interrupts the smooth decline in benzodiazepine concentrations, confuses your nervous system and disrupts the process of learning to cope without drugs, which is an essential part of the adaptation to withdrawal. If the withdrawal is slow enough, 'escape pills' should not be necessary.

2. Switching to a long-acting benzodiazepine

For people withdrawing from potent, short-acting drugs, such as Ativan, it is advisable, in fact imperative, to switch to a long-acting, slowly metabolised benzodiazepine such as diazepam.

Diazepam (Valium) is one of the most slowly eliminated of the benzodiazepines. It has a half-life, in your system, of up to 200 hours, which means that the blood level for each dose falls by only half in about 8.3 days. Slow elimination of diazepam allows a smooth, gradual fall in blood level, allowing the body to adjust slowly to a decreasing concentration of the benzodiazepines in your system. The switchover process needs to be carried out gradually, usually in stepwise fashion, substituting one dose at a time. The schedules in *The Ashton Manual* suggest dosage reductions occur every week or two, but each person should determine the most comfortable rate for himself or herself.

Another factor to bear in mind is that the various benzodiazepines, though broadly similar, have slightly different profiles of action.

For example, lorazepam (Ativan), which I was taking, seems to have less hypnotic activity than diazepam (probably because it is shorter acting).

Thus, if someone on 2mg Ativan three times a day is directly switched to 60mg diazepam (the equivalent dose for anxiety), he or she is liable to become extremely sleepy, but if they are switched suddenly onto a much smaller dose of diazepam, they will probably get withdrawal symptoms.

Making the changeover, one dose (or part of a dose) at a time to Valium avoids this difficulty and helps to find the equivalent dosage for that individual. It is also helpful to make the first substitution in the night-time dose, and the substitution may not always need to be complete.

For example, if your evening dose was 2mg Ativan, this could, in some cases, be changed down to 1mg Ativan plus 8mg diazepam combination. A full substitution for the dropped 1mg of Ativan would have been 10mg diazepam. However, the patient may sleep well on this combination and he will have already made a dosage reduction — a first step in withdrawal.

A third important practical factor is the available dosage formulations of the various benzodiazepines. In withdrawal, you'll need a long-acting drug, which can be reduced in very small steps. Diazepam (Valium) is the only benzodiazepine that is ideal for this purpose since it comes in 2mg tablets, which are scored down the middle and easily halved into 1mg doses. By contrast, the smallest available tablet of lorazepam (Ativan) is 0.5mg (equivalent to 5mg diazepam).

Some doctors in the US apparently switch patients onto clonazepam (Klonopin, Rivotril in Canada), believing that it will be easier to withdraw from than alprazolam (Xanax) or lorazepam (Ativan) because it is more slowly eliminated.

However, according to reliable sources, Klonopin is far from ideal for this purpose. It is an extremely potent drug, is eliminated much faster than diazepam and the smallest available tablet in the US, as I understand it, is 0.5mg (equivalent to 10mg diazepam) and 0.25mg in Canada (equivalent to 5mg Valium).

It is difficult with this drug to achieve a smooth, slow fall in blood concentration, and there is some evidence that withdrawal is particularly difficult from high-potency benzodiazepines, including Klonopin.

Because the benzo I was hooked on was Ativan (lorazepam), I'll use that as the basis for my advice in this book, but there are many charts of variations available for you online at *The Ashton Manual*, including the preceding information, to match the drug you're taking to the right withdrawal programme, so Google that and find the chart to match your drug. (And note that there are **two Ativan**

charts at *The Ashton Manual.* The example in this book is for 3mg daily but there is a 6mg daily chart also available.)

Here is more information to point you in the right direction:

Professor C. Heather Ashton's book, Benzodiazepines: How They Work and How to Withdraw, *also known as* The Ashton Manual, *is available at http://www.benzo.org.uk/manual/index.htm where it may be printed out directly from the computer. Hard copies of the book may be purchased at http://www.benzo.org.uk/bzmono.htm#order.*

Her paper entitled 'Reasons for a Diazepam (Valium) Taper' may be found at http://www.benzo.org.uk/ashvtaper.htm.

The Ashton Method is also, as far as I know, the only benzodiazepine discontinuation protocol that is based upon both rigorous scientific research as well as actual clinical experience, so I suggest you make that your 'go to' place for safe, well-researched in-depth information and treat with caution everything else you find on the 'net. I reiterate that most of the specific information in this final section of my book is based on Professor Ashton's manual, which she has authorised me to use, but also interpreted through the lens of my own personal experience.

3. Designing and following the withdrawal schedule

When switching over to diazepam, substitute one dose at a time (usually starting with the evening or night-time dose), then replace the other doses, one by one, at intervals of a few days or a week. Unless you are starting from very large doses, there is no need to aim for a reduction at this stage;

simply aim for an approximately equivalent dosage. When you have done this, you can start reducing the diazepam slowly.

Bear in mind, at this stage, you are only preparing for total withdrawal, which is some weeks away, so you will experience no problems or anxiety during the cross-over phase from your brand of benzo to the tapering equivalent of diazepam (Valium).

If, however, you are on a high dose, such as 6mg alprazolam (equivalent to 120mg diazepam), you may need to undertake some reduction while switching over, and may need to switch only part of the dosage at a time. The aim is to find a dose of diazepam that largely prevents withdrawal symptoms but is not so excessive as to make you sleepy.

Diazepam is very slowly eliminated and needs only, at most, twice-daily administration to achieve smooth blood concentrations. If you are currently taking benzodiazepines three or four times a day, it is advisable to space out your dosage to twice daily once you are on Valium. The less often you take tablets, the less your day will revolve around your medication.

The larger the dose you are taking initially, the greater the size can be of each dose reduction. You could aim at reducing dosage by up to one tenth at each decrement.

For example, if you are taking 40mg diazepam equivalent, you could reduce at first by 2–4mg every week or two. When you are down to 20mg, reductions could be 1–2mg weekly or fortnightly. When you are down to 10mg, 1mg reductions are probably indicated. From 5mg diazepam, some people prefer to reduce by 0.5mg every week or two.

It's up to you. It's yours to control and never let anyone try to divert or remove your control of what you're endeavouring to achieve, without qualification. (Softly, softly, catchee monkey — off your back!)

The Withdrawal Chart

Here is the chart that I wish I'd had access to when I started self-detox and that I should've followed during my tapering as it was Ativan that I was attempting to escape from. But despite my best efforts, I was unable to locate any such information in the nineties when I took the plunge.

Withdrawal Chart
Withdrawal from lorazepam (Ativan)
3mg daily with diazepam (Valium) substitution
(3mg lorazepam is approximately equivalent to 30mg diazepam)

	Morning	Midday/ Afternoon	Evening/ Night	Daily Diazepam Equivalent
Starting dosage	lorazepam 1 mg	lorazepam 1 mg	lorazepam 1 mg	30mg
Stage 1 (1 week)	lorazepam 1 mg	lorazepam 1 mg	lorazepam 0.5mg diazepam 5mg	30mg
Stage 2 (1 week)	lorazepam 0.5mg diazepam 5mg	lorazepam 1 mg	lorazepam 0.5mg diazepam 5mg	30mg
Stage 3 (1 week)	lorazepam 0.5mg diazepam 5mg	lorazepam 0.5mg diazepam 5mg	lorazepam 0.5mg diazepam 5mg	30mg
Stage 4 (1 week)	lorazepam 0.5mg diazepam 5mg	lorazepam 0.5mg diazepam 5mg	Stop lorazepam diazepam 10mg	30mg
Stage 5 (1 week)	Stop lorazepam diazepam 10mg	lorazepam 0.5mg diazepam 5mg	diazepam 10mg	30mg
Stage 6 (1 week)	diazepam 10mg	Stop lorazepam diazepam 10mg	diazepam 10mg	30mg
Stage 7 (1-2 weeks)	diazepam 10mg	diazepam 8mg	diazepam 10mg	28mg

Stage				
Stage 8 (1-2 weeks)	diazepam 8mg	diazepam 8mg	diazepam 10mg	26mg
Stage 9 (1-2 weeks)	diazepam 8mg	diazepam 6mg	diazepam 10mg	24mg
Stage 10 (1-2 weeks)	diazepam 6mg	diazepam 6mg	diazepam 10mg	22mg
Stage 11 (1-2 weeks)	diazepam 6mg	diazepam 4mg	diazepam 10mg	20mg
Stage 12 (1-2 weeks)	diazepam 6mg	diazepam 2mg	diazepam 10mg	18mg
Stage 13 (1-2 weeks)	diazepam 6mg	Stop diazepam	diazepam 10mg	16mg
Stage 14 (1-2 weeks)	diazepam 5mg	–	diazepam 10mg	15mg
Stage 15 (1-2 weeks)	diazepam 4mg	–	diazepam 10mg	14mg
Stage 16 (1-2 weeks)	diazepam 3mg	–	diazepam 10mg	13mg
Stage 17 (1-2 weeks)	diazepam 2mg	–	diazepam 10mg	12mg
Stage 18 (1-2 weeks)	diazepam 1mg	–	diazepam 10mg	11mg
Stage 19 (1-2 weeks)	Stop diazepam	–	diazepam 10mg	10mg

Source: *The Ashton Manual*: http://www.benzo.org.uk/manual/bzsched.htm

The chart looks straightforward as long as you stick to it to the best of your ability. **You will note that this is an**

Ativan withdrawal chart. There are other charts for different benzos and dosages available online at the *Ashton Manual.*

http://www.benzo.org.uk/manual/bzsched.htm

If you don't feel comfortable at the beginning, there is no need to draw up your withdrawal schedule right up to the end.

It is usually sensible to plan the first few weeks and then review it and, if necessary, amend your schedule according to your progress. Some people like to give their ongoing planned schedule to their trusted doctor, who has committed to be with you every step of the way.

Again, don't be a slave and accept just any doctor to 'ride shotgun' with you over the coming months of withdrawal. If you can't find a sympathetic one, just keep looking until you find a friendly professional that you're comfortable with before you enter the process of withdrawal. There is no hurry. Take your time and do it right.

Prepare your doctor to be flexible and to be ready for your schedule to be adjusted to a slower (or faster) pace at any time.

To the best of your ability and sanity, never, ever go backwards. You can stand still at a certain stage in your schedule and have a vacation from further withdrawal for a few weeks if circumstances change (for instance, if there is a family crisis), but try to avoid *ever* increasing the dosage again. You don't want to go back over ground you have already covered.

Do not become obsessed with your withdrawal schedule and let it rule your day. Let it just become a normal way of life for the next few months. Okay, you are withdrawing from your benzodiazepines; so are many others around the world at the same time as you. It's no big deal. Don't overthink it.

Avoid compensating for benzodiazepines by increasing your intake of alcohol, cannabis or non-prescription drugs. Occasionally, your doctor may suggest other drugs for particular symptoms. (Short-term, low-dosage beta-blockers of 25mg can be useful but only to cover a stressful occasion.)

Most addicts coming off any drug are inveterate smokers. If you're one of those, then allow yourself the luxury of having that one addiction during the drug withdrawal process.

Chances are that once you get clean, you'll want to dump the smokes anyway.

Lack of sleep in the early stages and in emotional withdrawal stage two is unavoidable and comes with the territory, but you will survive. I did!

The level of endurance of the human mind has never been tested, but no matter how bad your sleep patterns are, do not be tempted to take the sleeping tablets zolpidem (Ambien), zopiclone (Zimovane, Imovane) or zaleplon (Sonata), as they have the same actions as benzodiazepines and interfere with your sleep architecture.

Personally, I have found the natural hormone Melatonin 300 micrograms (mcg) very useful for getting to sleep. It is prescription only in a lot of countries, but easily available online. It is not a drug and is commonly used for jet lag, as it acts on the circadian rhythms emanating from the pituitary gland in the base of the brain.

A government survey published in 2016 found that 3.1 million Americans, 1.3% of the population, take melatonin supplements for jet lag and other sleep problems. Its use has more than doubled in the US between 2007 and 2012. I recommend it.

47

Stepping into freedom

Okay, that dreaded moment has arrived when you get down to your last tablet. Well done, you, for reaching this point. Stopping the last few milligrams is often viewed as particularly difficult. This is mainly due to fear of how you will cope without any drug at all. In fact, the final parting is surprisingly easy. People are usually delighted by the new sense of freedom gained and say that 'it's like the sun coming up again in their life'. Here's something to make you happy and relieved! The *last* 1mg or 0.5mg diazepam per day, which you are taking at the end of your schedule, is having very little effect on you, apart from keeping the dependence going.

Please do not be tempted to spin out the withdrawal to a ridiculously slow rate towards the end (such as 0.25mg each month). You've come this far so don't linger on that last 10mg diazepam. Drop it down as quickly as possible and then you're free! Take the plunge when you reach 0.5mg daily; full recovery cannot begin until you have got off your tablets completely.

Some people, after completing withdrawal, like to carry around a few tablets with them for security 'just in case', but find that they rarely, if ever, use them. This is ridiculous, silly and not advisable. You know deep in yourself it's all or nothing and having a backup pill is just admitting that you aren't in control of the process. You'll make it if you remain strong and staunch. After all, you're the one that stands to gain everything once you're free of the curse of the benzo devil!

If for any reason you do not (or did not) succeed at your first attempt at benzodiazepine withdrawal, don't beat yourself up. You can always try again. They say that most smokers make seven or eight attempts before they finally give up cigarettes. However, the good news is that most long-term benzodiazepine users are successful after their first attempt. Those who need a second try have usually been withdrawn too quickly the first time around. A slow and steady benzodiazepine withdrawal, with you in control, is nearly always successful.

48

Long-term effects of benzodiazepines

One mechanism that might be involved in the long-term (and possibly permanent) effects of benzodiazepines is an alteration in the activity of benzodiazepine receptors in the brain's GABA neurons. These receptors down-regulate (become fewer) as tolerance to benzodiazepines develop with chronic, long-term use.

Such down-regulation is a homeostatic response of the body to the constant presence of the drugs. Since benzodiazepines themselves enhance the actions of GABA, extra benzodiazepine receptors are no longer needed; so many are, in effect, discarded by the brain chemistry.

These down-regulated receptors are absorbed into neurons where, over time, they undergo various changes, including alterations in gene expression. When these receptors are slowly reinstated, after drug withdrawal, they may return in a slightly altered form.

They may not be quite so efficient as before in increasing the actions of GABA, the natural 'calming' neurotransmitter. As a result, the brain may be generally less sensitive to GABA and the individual is left with heightened central nervous system excitability and increased sensitivity to stress. Molecular biologists point out that changes in gene expression can be very slow, or even unable, to reverse.

Some people appear to be naturally more prone to anxiety than others. Brain imaging and pharmacological studies have shown that there is a decreased density (decreased numbers) and sub-sensitivity of brain. GABA/benzodiazepine receptors can be naturally fewer in people with generalised anxiety disorder or panic disorder and in patients with tinnitus, even if they have never been treated with benzodiazepines.

Perhaps these individuals with genetically fewer GABA/benzodiazepine receptors are those more likely to experience long-term effects of benzodiazepines' protracted symptoms after withdrawal and apparent recurrence of withdrawal symptoms, but such people are a very small minority.

49

Recurrence of symptoms after successful withdrawal

Half the modern drugs could well be thrown out the window, except that the birds might eat them.
— Martin Henry Fischer

It is not unusual to experience recurrence of apparent benzodiazepine withdrawal symptoms years after a successful withdrawal and you've returned to full, normal health. However, according to Professor Ashton, writing in the 2004 edition of *Comprehensive Handbook of Drug & Alcohol Addiction*, 85–95% of those getting off benzos do not have related problems of any significance once the use of the drug has been terminated.

The pattern of symptoms is unique to the individual, depending on his or her physical and psychological makeup, and, no doubt, on the innate density of his/her benzodiazepine GABA receptors. The experience of benzodiazepine withdrawal is deeply etched into the mind and memory bank of those who have been through it, and is actually physically present in the strength and connections of their neural synapses, as all memories are.

These recurrent symptoms are all signs of GABA under-activity, with its accompanying increased output of excitatory neurotransmitters resulting in a hyperactive, hypersensitive central nervous system. The mechanism is exactly the same as that of benzodiazepine withdrawal, which is why the symptoms are the same.

In nearly every case of apparent recurrence, the precipitating cause for the return of symptoms turns out, on close inspection, to be an increase in environmental stress. They can come (and go) sporadically but though they may hang around till you calm down from whatever it is that is stressing you, they do pass and vanish again for a long period of time. Ride it like a bad wave as, like all waves, they fizzle out as they roll up the beach of your life! It's an anxious world we all live in.

The trigger may be a new stress or worry which may be unrecognised, so that in the very unlikely event of the return of symptoms, it seems to occur out of the blue. Contributing factors can be an infection, surgery, dental problems, work problems, fatigue, bereavement, family problems, loss of sleep, adverse reaction to a drug, change of environment — almost anything. It may also be that with increasing age and long-term worries, the brain simply gets less efficient at coping with stress. However, this can be compensated for by research that clearly shows we get less anxious naturally, as we get older (and wiser).

In addition, there may still be some lingering, old disturbing worries / thoughts / memories that have been buried in the unconscious mind but are resurfacing now, because the brain has not been able to deal with them adequately in the past, due to the chemical blanket of whatever drug you've been taking for all that time.

This is where new, learned techniques like meditation and yoga, etc. are extremely helpful in calming your approach to stress. We all experience stress. That person next to you on the train looks so relaxed and calm, right? But inside their monkey mind they're freaking out about how to pay the mortgage, does my wife really love me and am I going to lose my job? Everybody is dampening down his or her inner hysteria in this high-powered world, so just relax and don't sweat the small stuff!

After complete recovery, you may find over the years that your tolerance to everyday drugs, for whatever condition, seems to spin you out or react adversely above what would be expected. It is not clear why many people report experiencing adverse effects from new drugs, or drugs they have tolerated before taking benzodiazepines. The drugs involved are so disparate — from skin ointments to eye drops to local anaesthetics to antidepressants, steroids and many others — that it is difficult to attribute these reactions to metabolic effects, allergies or other known effects.

Presumably the general hypersensitivity of the nervous system magnifies the reaction to any foreign substances, but no clear explanation has yet emerged. An exception is quinolone antibiotics, which displace benzodiazepines from their binding sites and, according to Professor Ashton, should not be taken by patients on, or recently on, benzodiazepines.

There is no evidence that nutritional supplements such as vitamins, minerals, amino acids, etc. are particularly helpful in benzodiazepine withdrawal unless the process has left you severely rundown from the stress and low diet. Excessive doses of some can be toxic and others may even contain benzo-like substances that have the same adverse effects as benzodiazepines themselves. Nor is there any evidence that suggests benzodiazepine withdrawal causes vitamin, mineral or other deficiencies.

Personally, I find the herbal tablet, St John's wort effective as a mood stabiliser and vitamin D, magnesium and zinc supplements to be useful, but there is nothing in the supplement world, despite what claims are made online, that can give you a guaranteed sense of calm, any more than a good meal or some satisfying sex.

However, there is a very strong developing argument for changing your daily diet from junk food, fizzy drinks, etc. to what is known as 'happy foods' (Google it). These include a lot of green vegetables and more importantly the daily inclusion of probiotics in your diet. We have two 'brains' and one is in the stomach as well as the head, so if you have healthy gut flora, science has shown that it affects your mental state of mind, including anxiety. Probiotics can be found in yoghurt or in capsule form from any health shop.

The Western diet typically has too few brain-essential nutrients such as B-group vitamins, vitamin D3, zinc, magnesium and omega-3 fish oil fatty acids. If you find a supplier of micro-nutrient capsules, then I would suggest that you definitely consider starting using them. The brain relies on a broad range of nutrients for the manufacture of good neurotransmitters such as serotonin, dopamine and adrenaline, which all will be out of balance when you're going through withdrawal. Research micro-nutrients online and you will see ample evidence of the benefits.

50

The end, the last tango

Well, here we are at the end. What a ride it's been. For me, writing my story has felt like acting in a movie about someone else, as I find it very hard to believe that I went through all that I did and survived.

Having done a lot of researching of a multitude of sources to put this book together, one thing I do now realise is that I personally dodged a bullet by sticking to the same daily intake of Ativan, as it seems that there's a huge amount of benzo addicts out there who are taking a multitude of benzo brands and, in some cases, a lot higher doses than I ever did, which would make it more complicated to withdraw from.

The main reason for writing this book is to help you by handing on my knowledge and experiences. It's that simple. To pass on to you the tightrope walk of the long and winding road from dependency to freedom and to, hopefully, point you in the right direction as to the protocols to follow when going through the withdrawal and tapering process. There are pockets of information available on the internet but there is no perfect answer to any of this and I don't profess to be a medical professional or man of science on the subject. I'm just a journeyman who has been through 'the fire' and made it to the other side, and all my book is meant to achieve is to give you the hope that you too can do the same, and be free.

I thank you for reading my story and I sincerely hope that it has motivated you to follow my path to freedom. If you wish to communicate further, go to the Facebook page 'The Benzo Devil' and we can go from there.

Plan your withdrawal strategy then take a long, delicious breath and jump in off the deep end of your life and don't stop 'swimming' till you reach the shallows. It will be worth it. You have my guarantee. Good luck.

References and links

The Ashton Manual, http://www.benzo.org.uk/manual/index.htm

Video: Limbic System, Introductory Overview, *Brain Mind Lecture 6,* Rhawn Joseph, Ph.D. BrainMind.com. https://youtu.be/T7nXiXQb2iM

Benzo Withdrawal: Part 1 Nervous System. https://youtu.be/89iAcGB-aYo

Benzo Withdrawal: Part 2 The Neuron. https://youtu.be/VJtNnTtbxjY

Benzo Withdrawal: Part 3 Neurotransmitters. https://youtu.be/0uJtGPDIpj0

Benzo Withdrawal: Part 4 GABA, GABAa Receptor, Benzos. https://youtu.be/QAUIThbiuFY

Benzo Withdrawal: Part 5 Brain on Benzos. https://youtu.be/S5T42_trA1A

Advocates against benzos:

- Dr Allen J Frances, former head of psychiatry at Princeton University, former chairman of the

Department of Psychiatry at Duke University School of Medicine, Chair of the DSM IV

- Professor Heather Ashton
- Professor Malcolm Lader OBE
- Psychiatrist Dr Peter Breggin
- *The Ashton Manual,* http://www.benzo.org.uk
- The Benzodiazepine Information Coalition, www.benzoinfo.com
- The Benzodiazepine Medical Disaster, https://vimeo.com/188181193
- As Prescribed documentary, http://www.asprescribedfilm.com/
- Letters from Generation RX, http://www.lettersfromgenerationrx.com/
- Benzo Buddies, www.benzobuddies.org
- Benzo-Wise and Recovery Experience (B-WaRE), https://www.facebook.com/groups/660273474151978/
- Benzodiazepine Recovery, https://www.facebook.com/groups/benzorecovery/
- Benzodiazepine Awareness and Legal Action, https://www.facebook.com/groups/benzoawareness/
- Beating Benzos, https://www.facebook.com/groups/Beatingbenzos/
- Benzo and 'GABA Drug' Use and Recovery Experiences (Medical professionals and benzo victims),

https://www.facebook.com/groups/
1486765754987409/

CME for Psychiatrists About Benzodiazepines.
https://youtu.be/SMzaxAo-sxI
Promo Video 1: World Benzodiazepine Awareness Day
2016. https://youtu.be/2X6ZFmo3VBY

Disclaimer

The material published in this book is for general information to the public. The author and publisher are not engaged in rendering medical, health, psychological advice or any other kind of personal or professional services. Most of the material contained in parts one to four of this book is based only on the author's personal experience and is opinion only.

The material should not be considered complete and does not cover all diseases, ailments, physical conditions or their treatment. The information about drugs contained in this book is general in nature. It does not cover all possible uses, actions, precautions, side effects, or interactions of the medicines mentioned. The material provided herein should not be used for diagnosing or treating a health problem or disease. It is not a substitute for professional care nor should it be used in place of a call or visit to a medical, health or other competent professional, nor is the information intended as medical advice for individual problems or for making an evaluation as to the risks and benefits of taking a particular drug.

The author does not assume responsibility for any inaccuracies or omissions or for consequences from use of material obtained in this book and the author specifically disclaims all responsibility for any liability, loss or risk, personal or otherwise, which may be incurred as a consequence, directly or indirectly, of the use and application of any of the material in this book.

It is suggested that readers consult other sources of information as well as obtain direct consultation with a physician when making decisions about their health care. If you have, or suspect you may have, a health problem, you should consult your professional health care provider. The material in this book is in no way intended to replace medical advice offered by physicians or a complete medical history and physical examination by a physician. In any event and before adopting any of the suggestions in this book or *The Ashton Manual* or drawing inferences from it, you should consult your professional health care provider.

IMPORTANT NOTICE

Any information given in this book should not be substituted for the advice of a physician **who is well informed** about benzodiazepine addiction and withdrawal. All information given here is therefore to be followed at your own risk. Abrupt cessation of benzodiazepines may be very dangerous. Always consult your prescriber if you are considering making any changes.

About the Author

R.W. Pharazyn has been involved in radio and media for 25 years both in his home country of New Zealand and Australia. He's best known as a former, top rating talkback radio host and 'rock jock' but has also been a successful newspaper publisher.

He swears that retirement is for fools and horses and instead chooses to use the term 'refocusing' when it comes to taking on new projects.

He loves wine, craft beer, good food, pretty women and Paris (not necessarily in that order). He is grateful to be alive.

You can contact the author via his Facebook Page: The Benzo Devil
https://www.facebook.com/benzodevil